Praise for the work of Meir Schneider

"I have been impressed with the work of Meir Schneider for many years, having personally seen improvements in patients' vision of those who have worked with him. The ability of the visual system to adapt and regain function is still full of mysteries. Through Meir's work, we are finding some of those mysteries to be realities."

> — August L. Reader III, MD, FACS, clinical professor of ophthalmology, California Pacific Medical Center

"Meir's method is effective as a complementary physical therapy for the eyes."

> — Emília Ritsuko Yasuoka Assad, ophthalmologist and acupuncturist

"Working with my patients has verified that many sight problems get better and heal by taking up the right habits. Meir presents us with a complete guide to do so. He helps us to regain our trust in the power we have over our vision and our lives. As he says in the book, 'We all can take the time. We just have to decide that we are worth the time and that the process is worth our while.'"

> — Amelia Salvador, ophthalmologist, Spain

"As an ophthalmologist, I always search for the best way to treat my patients. Based on the Bates Method, self-healing has complemented my practice in those cases where our traditional medicine has its limitations. The best treatment is the one that is directed to the patient's needs, and the best medicine is the one that uses all knowledge and not only a part of it. Traditional science and complementary medicine are tools that should be used together, focusing on a more holistic health concept."

> — Leonardo Verri Paulino, MD, ophthalmologist and anterior segment surgeon at ABC Medical School, Brazil

"It is wonderful how each new book by Meir Schneider provokes us to incorporate more and more of the self-healing principles into our lives."

> — Laercio Motoryn, MD, ophthalmologist and homeopath

"I had the pleasure to meet Meir Schneider and use his method when I was finishing my apprenticeship to become a Bachelor of Optometry in 2005. His holistic approach toward visual dysfunctions changed me forever as a professional. His concepts remain present in my appointments, therapies, and lens prescriptions. Meir's work invites us to naturally preserve our organism and to practice healthier visual habits in this very technological world."

— Fernando Nassif, optometrist with specialization in orthoptics and visual therapy

"The knowledge and application of the Self-Healing Method was very important to improve my practice as an ophthalmologist. The results attained by my patients and with my own vision are proof of the importance of the union of traditional medicine with complementary therapies. I thank Meir for being such a marvelous instrument for my personal and professional improvement."

— Ana Cecilia Gois Franco, ophthalmologist and anterior segment surgeon and naturopath, São Paulo, Brazil

"There are many kinds of patients, but those who get actively involved with their own healing process can surely go further. When I met Meir Schneider years ago, I started to apply some of his techniques to my work and was impressed by the results. We must imprint our will and optimism into everything we do, so we can go beyond it. Congratulations, Meir, for one more book that brings us simple yet useful lessons."

—Mauro Rabinovitch, MD, ophthalmologist Sao Paulo, Brazil

Vision for Life

Also by Meir Schneider

Movement for Self-Healing
The Handbook of Self-Healing
Self-Healing: My Life and Vision

Vision
FOR LIFE

10 Steps to
Natural Eyesight Improvement

REVISED EDITION

MEIR SCHNEIDER, PhD

North Atlantic Books
Berkeley, California

Published by
North Atlantic Books
Huichin, unceded Ohlone land
aka Berkeley, California

Cover photo © knikola/Shutterstock.com
Cover design by Howie Severson
Book design by Brad Greene

Printed in Canada

Vision for Life: 10 Steps to Natural Eyesight Improvement, Revised Edition is sponsored and published by North Atlantic Books, an educational nonprofit based in the unceded Ohlone land Huichin (*aka* Berkeley, CA) that collaborates with partners to develop cross-cultural perspectives; nurture holistic views of art, science, the humanities, and healing; and seed personal and global transformation by publishing work on the relationship of body, spirit, and nature.

North Atlantic Books' publications are distributed to the US trade and internationally by Penguin Random House Publisher Services. For further information, visit our website at www.northatlanticbooks.com.

MEDICAL DISCLAIMER: The following information is intended for general information purposes only. Individuals should always see their health care provider before administering any suggestions made in this book. Any application of the material set forth in the following pages is at the reader's discretion and is their sole responsibility.

Library of Congress Cataloging-in-Publication Data

The Library of Congress has cataloged the first edition as follows:
Schneider, Meir, 1954–
  Vision for life : ten steps to natural eyesight improvement / Meir Schneider.
     p. cm.
  Summary: "Presents ten simple steps to relieve eye strain, correct visionproblems, and improve eye health; includes a full range of restorative visionexercises"—Provided by publisher.
  ISBN-13: 978-1-58394-494-3
  ISBN-10: 1-58394-494-X
  1. Vision disorders—Treatment. 2. Visual training. 3. Orthoptics. 4. Bates method of orthoptics. 5. Eye—Diseases—Treatment. 6. Blindness—Genetic aspects. I. Title.
  RE992.O7S27 2012
  617.7'5—dc23
This edition ISBN-13; 978-1-62317-008-0 / ISBN-10: 1-62317-008-7

5 6 7 8 9 10 11 MQ 26 25 24 23 22

Contents

Foreword

Whoever has had the privilege to attend a lecture given by Meir Schneider knows that one does not passively listen to his work. The audience members are immediately treated as students and invited to perform exercises right there in the conference room. According to Meir, more important than talking about his method is experiencing it; theory is only valuable when implemented. We are beings with an incredible adaptive capacity, and so is his teaching: simple, direct, and transformative. It goes beyond the barrier of predefined concepts and comes with the assurance that we can walk away from the passiveness of our routine actions and into the freshness of new ones.

This book is a mirror of his way of teaching. The interactive and dynamic contents express the author's quality, moving us away from the apparent security of restrictive visual habits to experience new possibilities. Since he considers that we all can improve our vision naturally, this book is not destined only for those who have diagnosed visual dysfunctions; this is for all of us. As Meir always says, routine is the ultimate degenerative disease.

I first met Meir Schneider in 1992, at a conference for six hundred people in São Paulo, Brazil. He made such an impression on the audience that it became the perfect time for the first training course in that country. I took part in it, although I had no previous experience in the health area. To be a health professional was not a prerequisite for Meir, however. He wanted to keep his teaching open to whoever was up to working on themselves. This closer contact with the technique completely changed my way of relating to my body and my cognitive processes. Soon I started teaching others, thus complementing my learning experience. A few years later, already working as a fully trained therapist who specialized in visual education, I felt an urge to deepen my theoretical knowledge and went back to school to become an optometrist. This skill gave me better conditions under which to appreciate the grandeur of the method—Meir's great ability to bring complex theory into something that speaks to us. After all, theory tries to explain what we are. And Meir translates it with rare intelligence and generosity. There is no hidden material in his teaching; it is all there, at the reach of minds willing to experience themselves.

This book is much more than a guide to exercises; it is an invitation to transformation. Good reading.

— M. Fernanda Leite Ribeiro, optometrist and self-healing practitioner
   and instructor

Preface

The world may soon be faced with an epidemic of vision disorders, as hundreds of millions of humans who have been subjected to constant contact with computer screens, fluorescent lights, and excessively lit cities gradually enter old age. Tragically, although they seem adequately equipped to predict such a catastrophe, the existing medical establishment is not at all prepared to correctly address this epidemic. From my personal experience, I believe medical doctors often tend to suffer from their own form of myopia, a shortsighted attitude toward holistic approaches to body repair and maintenance.

In modern times, where culture has influenced our values for most of our lifetimes, we understand the importance in any successful endeavor of budgeting for repair and maintenance. If we intend to maintain the value and the beauty of any product or system throughout its lifespan, and to extend that lifespan for as long as possible, steps must be taken along the way to maintain the usefulness of all vital systems, and to correct any defects that develop along the way due to misuse, neglect, or accidental damage. Human beings need even more attention than machines in this respect; we need nurturing.

I am happy that people are beginning to wake up to this notion, and that a preventive, protective attitude has already begun working its way into the human psyche. Every day, more people pay closer attention to the food and beverages they consume, to the environment in which they live, and to establishing general healthy habits like physical exercise. But we still do not spend enough time addressing the health and well-being of our eyes. That is the purpose of *Vision for Life:* to help people maintain and repair their vision as a way to increase the length and quality of their lives.

It seems ironic to me that the scientific establishment might be to blame for the sorry condition in which we are finding ourselves. The success that optometry and ophthalmology professions have had in recent decades is largely to blame for our culture's laissez-faire attitude toward the health of our eyes. This has happened by correcting vision problems through prescriptive lenses and surgical technology without offering any alternative.

People often take it for granted that if something goes wrong with their vision, medical science will come to their rescue. And while this may be true in many cases, I am a firm believer that it is always better to prevent a disease in the first place rather than to simply wait for the system to break down in hopes that science will offer a solution. First of all, preventative medicine is cheaper! Compare twenty minutes a day of aerobic exercise, such as running along the beach or bicycling through the park, to the extreme cost of a surgical procedure to correct clogged arteries. Even factoring in the price of an expensive luxury gym membership and regular massages, the preventative approach is still far less expensive.

We must commit right now to creating a health regimen for our eyes, because the whole body is affected by eyestrain. The human eye was made to hunt, to scan the horizon, to look at birds, to look into the distance. It was designed to be engaged in a variety of circumstances, looking at different things at different distances and in different light. If we stare only at a computer screen all day under the same lighting, we lose the variation as well as the acuity. We lose the passion for looking and seeing the diversity of life around us. What then does this do to our bodies and to our energy levels?

So many people report that they feel exhausted in the middle of the day, that they need stimulants to revive them. We must remember that whatever we do with the eyes affects the whole body.

The habits that you will develop if you follow the exercises in *Vision for Life* can be the lifeline you need. You will reinvent your passion for life while protecting the vision you have and correcting the degenerative condition from which you suffer. Best of all, as with any kind of personal exercise regimen, these habits will impact your life in ways that transcend the utilitarian benefits of disease prevention.

Like the poet said, the eyes are the windows to the soul. By connecting with our vision, we connect with light and darkness, with nature, with our physical environment, and with each other in fundamental, simple, and beautiful ways. Going for a jog doesn't have to be just good physical exercise, it can also be a welcome relief for the mind. It is a way to reconnect with your neighborhood, to break out of your routine, and to expand your psychological comfort zone. And the same can be said of learning how to blink correctly, practicing the scrutiny of details, looking far into the distance, and nighttime walking.

Computers have certainly done much to advance the quality of life in our culture. Yet every year, as hundreds of millions more people world-wide incorporate computers into their routines, they expose their precious eyes to constant unnatural strain and poor lighting. By straining their central vision to stare blurry-eyed at the screen, people forget to utilize their peripheral vision. They forget to blink. They forget to breathe correctly. They scrunch their shoulders and tense their necks. They squint, trying to analyze digital data. And instead of using the natural human ability to scan for images, they simply sit and wait passively for the flood of constantly changing images to come to them. We must be proactive in taking care of our eyes in front of the computer in order to prevent vision problems and keep our eyes refreshed on a regular basis.

It is our joy and responsibility to personally make the effort to connect with nature and with our own human potential. We each must make the commitment to claim our heritage and our birthright, which is health, happiness, and a long-lasting, balanced, productive life. And it all starts with our eyes!

Our senses connect us intimately with each other, with our environment, and with ourselves, perhaps none so much as our sense of vision. When a person loses his or her vision, there is no end to what he or she will pay for a doctor to correct the situation. Sadly, however, many procedures performed on people's eyes today, including LASIK surgery, do more harm than good.

Compounding the problem even further is that many people's eyesight ratings are misdiagnosed at the optometrist's office because of the stress and nervousness people feel while they are having their eyes tested for glasses. Often, people are understandably stressed, and strain their vision out of fear that it may have declined. Their visual capacity on an average, relaxed day differs greatly from that when they are fearful and stressed. But when have you ever heard of an optometrist confronting this reality? When has your optometrist massaged your shoulders and asked you to breathe deeply before measuring your eyes? When has your ophthalmologist asked you to pray or meditate prior to measuring your eye pressure?

Most optometrists make no effort to test their patients' vision under normal, less stressful circumstances. And most people have no capacity to test their own vision when they are in a friendlier environment. Consequently, most people's glasses prescriptions are incorrectly based on stressed vision. The result is that the eyes, having no choice, learn to accommodate the incorrect prescription by weakening, adjusting gradually in the wrong direction toward worse, not better, vision. In fact, most optometrists don't even think stress relates to poor vision at all. The only way to adjust to a stronger prescription is to get the eyes weak enough that the prescription fits. And so the eyes slowly but surely get worse and worse. *Stress does decrease the strength of you vision (acuity).* Some people have a feeling of dizziness when they wear their new glasses because they are too strong for their eyes when they are not in a stressful setting, such as the optometrist's office. My personal experience in working with dozens of thousands of students and patients contradicts what these doctors think they know. Stress and poor vision do indeed go hand in hand.

So I advise my patients and students to sometimes take their lenses off while practicing the techniques I teach them, and I advise readers of this book to do the same. When you are in a safe environment, do the exercises periodically and always with your glasses off. It is no different than learning to walk again after a leg injury. If you never let go of the crutches, your legs can never regain their strength and improve to their full potential. Therefore, work out your eyes in the same ways you work out the rest of your body at the gym, but remember to do it with great relaxation.

The exercises in this book are intended to help you to create a basic, fundamentally healthy routine that you can incorporate into your life immediately. If enough of us practice these exercises diligently and work on improving vision throughout our lives, we can avoid the coming epidemic of cataracts, macular degeneration, and other degenerative conditions of the eyes that scientists predict are speeding toward our culture like a freight train.

Ask yourself what is in the medical establishment's best interest. Is it to help you to heal yourself with only an investment of time and self-healing work, or is it to find the quick fix that the average person is looking for in the form of a pill or surgery? I am not trying to be accusatory or conspiratorial. I am simply attempting to rephrase the wisdom of an old adage that says you should never ask a barber if you need a haircut. Never ask an optometrist if you need glasses, because in most instances if a person has his eyes examined and their vision is less than 20/20 the doctor will prescribe glasses to get you to see 20/20. It doesn't matter if you see 98 percent of 20/20 or 50 percent of 20/20 they will prescribe you corrective lenses because they do not believe you can improve your vision. But, if that doctor sent you home with exercises to strengthen your vision and relax your over stressed eyes you would very likely return the next year to find that you have returned to having 20/20. The medical establishment is so dependent on technology and chemicals that it has little incentive to embrace a simpler, less expensive, personal, holistic approach to vision maintenance and repair.

This book is my response to this serious problem, and it is also my attempt to give human beings an alternative to becoming the playthings of profit-driven, narrow-minded scientists who do not explore the whole truth. You are your own patient first. Heal yourself using the techniques in this book and other books like it. Seek the aid of chemicals and surgery only as a last resort, or in the most serious of situations.

For those of you who have perfect vision, or even better than perfect vision, now is the time to incorporate simple habits into your life, ensuring that your extraordinary vision will be maintained for as much of your life as possible. To that end, I have attempted to give you a lifetime of acquired knowledge all in one volume. Make your vision a central priority by devoting as much time as possible to the application of this book's principles. It is my dream that everyone will integrate my work into their own personal vision for life.

My unrestricted California driver's license.

Introduction

At one time, this book was to be titled *From Blindness to Vision,* because I was born blind but, through years of effort and exploration, have taught myself to see. Today, because of this miracle, I can read, write, and drive a car. The idea behind the original title was that my seemingly miraculous progression from blindness to sight would signal to readers that within this book are the resources anyone can use to improve their vision, regardless of their current situation.

In reality, I believe the great majority of this book's readers will not be those who are declared, as I was, legally blind. Rather, they will be people from all different points on the continuum of vision, including some with "perfect" vision who want to keep it or even build on it. As dramatic as our first title sounded, we wanted to make certain that readers would not mistake this for a handbook only for the blind or severely visually impaired. We gave up our attention-grabbing idea, and looked for another title.

Nonetheless, my personal experience in overcoming blindness remains at the core of this work. To anyone who doubts that improving his or her vision is possible, my story is a true testament to hope. It was therefore important to describe briefly just how this transformation happened. A detailed account of my life can be found in my earlier book, *Movement for Self-Healing,* which chronologically addresses the physical challenges I faced as well as the long series of steps, discoveries, and exercises I underwent to overcome them.

Now I wish to summarize this same process with more emphasis on the psychological aspect. These emotional and spiritual challenges were central to the process of my learning to see. The key obstacles that you, the reader, will face—whether you're legally blind or have the eagle eyes of an Air Force fighter pilot—will be similar to mine, even though the circumstances of our lives probably differ dramatically. The central challenge is for you to make a commitment to invest the necessary time to improve your vision and to expand your world.

It was difficult enough for me to do this in the 1970s in Israel, even with the burning, intrinsic motivation to rid myself of my blindness. For modern readers, to make this kind of dedication of time in our hectic, hyper era may seem impossible. Yet a commitment to doing it can pay off in two extraordinary ways: you will improve your vision while opening up your life.

Free yourself from the grip of a stressful routine. The amount of time and dedication I have devoted to improving my vision was extreme compared to what most people need, but that is exactly the point. Dedicate as much time as possible to these exercises, and remember that although your life may seem busy, making your vision a central priority is of the utmost importance.

List of Materials for Getting Started

- 4 pieces of dark construction paper cut 2 by 2 inches, 2 by 5 inches, 2 by 7 inches, and 2 by 9 inches
- masking tape
- tennis balls: at least two, preferably used; your local tennis club would most likely give you a few
- obstruction glasses (described in step 8 in chapter 2)*
- red and green glasses*
- red pencil or pen (use a red felt-tip pen if vision loss is extreme)
- plain white copy paper
- small flashlight with red bulb or red tape over the lens
- red and green playing cards (optional)*
- 10-foot and 20-foot eye charts (charts included in this book)*
- flashing lights (when working with severe vision loss)*
- glow-in-the-dark ball*
- beads on a string*
- pinhole glasses (optional)*
- shifter

*These items can often be made at home from materials found locally, but you can also order them from the School for Self-Healing (www .self-healing.org). Email the School For Self-Healing at officemanager @self-healing.org to order or if you have any questions.

Figure 1.1. My father, Abraham, mother, Eda, and me, age five, looking and seeing next to nothing.

Chapter 1

Healing Myself of Blindness

I was born in the Stalinist Soviet Union under difficult circumstances. My father was involved in an illegal business, taking and printing photographs for churches. This work could have resulted in his being sent to Siberia for twenty years. Furthermore, both my parents were deaf.

My grandparents on my father's side were opposed to another child coming into the family but could not stop my parents from bringing one. So some people say that I was a mistake. But my parents were very happy that I was born. At first, it was my paternal grandfather who noticed that something was wrong with my eyes. After an examination by doctors, it was revealed that I had been born with cataracts. Although many people develop cataracts later in life, very few are born with them. I was, for all practical purposes, born blind. One can ask why I was born with cataracts because my mother did not have rubella, which is known to be a cause. Only one out of twenty thousand infants are ever born with cataracts. I've heard the opinion that, because my father had an illegal laboratory—which he was hiding—and because I was a very weak infant, several times at the brink of death from undiagnosed illnesses, it could have been a chemical imbalance that caused my cataracts. Furthermore, cataracts are considered to be genetic. But I was the anomaly in my family. And, eventually, my kids inherited my gene. Or was it the psychological reason that there was great resistance to a new child being born in the family? Is it even possible for infants to carry the conflict within families and then be born with symptoms related to the conflict? When a cataract grows, it creates opacity, and unlike the cases of my own kids, my childhood surgeries were never successful. Were the difficulties in my family life therefore a contributing element to my condition?

In search of a better life for all of us, my family decided to flee the Soviet Union and relocate to the new country of Israel. During this time of transition for my family, five surgeries were performed on my eyes. The first, done in Poland on our way to Western Europe, was unsuccessful. The other four surgeries—all performed in Israel—scarred my lenses to the point that 99 percent of them was scar tissue, effectively preventing almost all light from getting through. As a result, I was issued a Blind Certificate by the state of Israel, and most people in my life had resigned themselves to the idea that I would never be able to see.

Figure 1.2. Blind Certificate: the state of Israel declaring me permanently blind.

I was raised reading Braille, although I attended a standard school with normal-sighted children. I experienced much loneliness and isolation because of this situation. What do you do when you are blind, surrounded by normal-sighted people, and your parents communicate mostly with sign language that you cannot see?

In Israel at that time, the concept of inclusion of legally blind kids in a normal school was novel; educators went to the United States and brought it back as a new idea. Until then, blind kids were schooled only at a special institution in Jerusalem, learning with other blind kids. I agreed with the idea of inclusion and was included by the fact that general study was from 8 a.m. to noon with most of the other kids, and mine was later on, from noon to 2 p.m., in a special place called the Braille Classroom. So instead of learning just with blind kids, I first integrated with other kids, and then I went to mentoring with the Braille teachers. Some of the Braille teachers were impatient and, to some extent, abusive. Nevertheless, it was a fantastic concept, especially in my case, because not only did I want to integrate, I also wanted to be one of the other kids. That was probably the beginning of my motivation to move forward and away from the limited vision I had. I kept working, and while the progress was slow, it felt like my world changed completely.

My father, who was very interested in current events, often wanted me to listen to the radio and to explain to him what was happening around the world. He would have me listen to the news and repeat it to him, which confused me at first. I didn't understand why he always lifted my head up when I tried to tell him what I had heard. I later realized it was because he wanted to read my lips. But how would I know that reading lips was so important when I couldn't even see lips moving? This tragic comedy more or less captures the early days of my life. I was surrounded by confusion, frustration, and struggle. But I was also learning that there are many ways to overcome the challenges people face due to the circumstances of their lives.

It was obvious to me that my parents loved me. Still, our life was marked by fear and insecurity, having escaped the repressions of the Soviet Union, only to move to the young state of Israel, which was ravaged with war. Because of their deafness, my parents could not study Hebrew, which was so different from the Russian they had spoken before. Additionally, my maternal grandparents lost all the money they had brought with them from the Soviet Union in bad investments in Israel. Yet through it all, my grandmother steadfastly believed in me and was able to find ways to help me. She stayed with me in hospital beds after surgeries, when I was traumatized and feeling insecure from hearing many other kids crying.

Other members of my family believed that I should depend on social services. Although I didn't mind asking for money from my family, somehow I did not want to take it from the government. It was a deep instinct, the origin of which I understood later on as I matured. It is easy for a person who receives help from the government, as many with disabilities do, to develop a poor self-image as being needy or pitiful; it comes automatically, like it or not. But when you do not rely on that help, the image you have of yourself becomes stronger, and you are forced to become self-sufficient.

I was determined not to have the stigma of being a blind person. That basic resolve was the beginning of my transition and change, without which I would not have gotten to where I am today. As a response to the lack of security and uncertainty that filled my early life, I grew a sense of commitment. Kids often did not want to play with me. Girls would not dance with me at parties. I sometimes became lonely. But I understood the choice was with me to be depressed or to be happy.

So, I escaped into my Braille books. With my books, I was in a different world and would read for hours on end. Even when my mother said, "Time to sleep; lights out," I would just hide the books under my bed. Due to my mother's deafness, she could not hear me. Although our walls were thin, as soon as the lights were out and I knew that she couldn't see me anymore, I pulled out my books again and kept reading. Most of the time, I was able to sneak in a couple of hours of reading without anyone noticing.

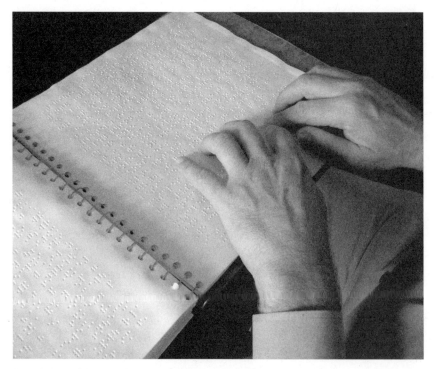

Figure 1.3. As of the seventh grade, I was the fastest Braille reader in Israel.

Whenever more of my Braille books arrived at the post office, I would hurry to pick them up. The books were huge. I was something to marvel at, a small kid carrying a very large school bag on my back, tied and strapped to my shoulders, with a Braille typewriter squeezed under one arm, while the other arm held a sack of Braille books. More than once, the typewriter fell and broke, and we had to pay to get it repaired. My father always resented the cost, and I felt guilty about having let the typewriter fall.

Slowly but surely, my muscles built up. Many a passerby felt I was engaged in too much lifting and carrying. But that lifting, in many ways, formed my character. I imagined that, one day, something would liberate me from my blindness, and I acted by it.

I went from doctor to doctor on my own. I struggled against the resentment of the other children in school who thought I was receiving too much special treatment. They resented the fact that they had to explain to me what was on the blackboard. And I agreed with them; I wanted to be able to see the blackboard with my own eyes. I wanted to work on my own. I even had teachers that were mean to me because they felt I was not behaving right. They believed a blind kid was supposed to be submissive and passive—something I never was and most likely never would be.

I desperately wanted to be liberated from my condition. But all the doctors told me there was nothing I could do, that legal blindness was going to be my life, and that my vision would never be more than 0.5 percent without glasses, nor more than 4 or 5 percent with glasses. They said to accept the sight I had, and that I should be happy with it. Those were nice words, but they did not work for me.

Discovering the Bates Method

My father was openly upset at the fact that his deafness prevented him from succeeding in life. My mother also felt like she was put down by the hearing world. I understood the prejudice they had experienced but, nonetheless, felt I had a bright future, though I did not know what it was.

Then one day, I met another young boy, named Jacob, who had dropped out of high school. He showed me eye exercises based on something called the Bates Method. I learned the eye exercises and started to work with them diligently.

To my amazement, as I practiced the Bates Method and experienced improvement, I received more complaints than ever from the authority figures in my life. You see, part of my practice was to look from detail to detail; the purpose of this exercise was to stop my brain from being lazy. But my geography teacher would get upset as I moved my eyes from one bell to the other, looking at the details during class. She went all the way to the vice principal. Thankfully, the vice principal heard my case and told her that the exercises may help me, and that they did not disturb my ability to listen to her lessons.

My Bible teacher was upset that, when my class sat in the yard reading biblical verses, I would close my eyes and face the sun, moving my head from side to side. When I faced the sun, my pupils would contract; when I moved my head to the side, my pupils would expand. My teacher said that it bothered him to see me moving my head from side to side, even though he recognized that I understood everything he was saying. He said that, even though I was the best student in the class, I should stop doing the sunning because it bothered him.

Figure 1.4. With these glasses, I was able to read the largest letter on the eye chart from a distance of five feet (20/800).

Despite these reactions, I persisted. My retina started to wake up to light, and that was my vehicle to removing the thick, heavy, dark glasses that had made the world dimmer for me. My mother was upset with the fact that I would run, ten times a day, up to the roof to do sunning. She said, "You're taking time out from your homework." Then she was upset that I would for sit three hours a day and do palming, an exercise to rest my eyes and stop them from moving involuntarily.

In short, I encountered so much resistance to what I did that I didn't even know it was possible to attempt change without facing resistance. When everybody resists you, not only does difficulty come in doing the exercises, but it also comes in dealing with the fact that your family, friends, teachers, and even neighbors oppose your efforts. Still, I persisted.

Within three months, I was able to see print. And not with a correction of 38 diopters, which is a microscope lens, but with a correction of 20 diopters, which is simply a very thick lens. Headaches that had plagued me all my life disappeared within six months.

Seeing the Light

Within a year of practicing the Bates Method, I was able to see regular letters. I'll never forget the day I was doing the sunning exercise on a roof, and looking at sharp black letters printed on white paper. I placed the paper at the tip of my nose. For the very first time in my life, at the age of seventeen and a half, I could see the printed word without magnification. This success took such a huge effort that I threw up. Again, I sunned and palmed and threw up until I saw another letter, then another. Soon, I heard loud voices in argument. It was the neighbors downstairs accusing each other of creating a mess on the windows. I hadn't realized that each time I threw up it was over their windows. So I went downstairs and told them what had happened. Instead of being angry with me, they were amazed at my honesty. I could have ignored my deeds, but I didn't. I was proud of the fact that I could finally see a letter. I honed my process and, within three months, could see multiple letters by putting the print right in front of my nose.

From then on, I continued to work. People were surprised that instead of just feeling my way down the road, I could literally see the road. Instead of not recognizing them, I started to know their faces. One neighbor was actually upset that I could recognize her. "What's wrong?" she would ask. "You're the blind person in the neighborhood. How can you see us? What have you done? What's going on?" It was amazing. I had taken away from her the feeling of security that resulted from knowing what was going on in the neighborhood. It was almost as if she felt the world she knew had been taken away. Here is the blind kid looking at everyone and actually seeing them. I was used to resistance, but was pleasantly surprised by the first voices of admiration I received.

My diligence continued. I looked from detail to detail. People finally accepted that I could see and recognize them, so my status soon changed from being one who was nearly blind to one who was nearly sighted. I kept working despite the fact that my progress was slow.

A landmark came when Jacob, my instructor of vision improvement, told me I no longer had astigmatism. Don't ask me how he knew, but when I went to the ophthalmologist in the public clinic, she was shocked. She said to me, "I don't know how it happened, but you don't have astigmatism. You don't need the cylinders anymore." I was not surprised to hear this.

It was at this time that I was taught the connection between the health of my eyes and that of the rest of my physical body through my work with Miriam, my grandmother's librarian, who taught me a series of exercises to improve my body. I began to practice movement techniques and learned that movement is life. I knew Miriam through an exchange of books between her and my grandmother and because she had introduced me to Jacob in the first place. He was also the person who read two books on the Bates Method: Aldous Huxley's *The Art of Seeing* and Harold Peppard's *Sight Without Glasses,* which were translated into Hebrew but went out of print rather quickly. Jacob improved his vision and overcame nearsightedness from 5.5 diopters to no glasses—and he was a high school dropout. My grandmother influenced me to meet him and was always behind me, even when she resisted because I devoted so much to work with my eyes, and later on to helping others work with theirs. Her love, as well as my mother's, was the reason I was able to help myself, and it made a big difference in my motivation.

Whenever circumstances block possibilities of improvement, there are always other possibilities that can help you move forward. I learned from experience that the human body is capable of improving and healing itself. We forget that we have the potential to improve our vision. The world is so engaged in the myth that poor eyesight cannot improve, especially in a case like mine, that it is difficult to imagine a story like mine being true.

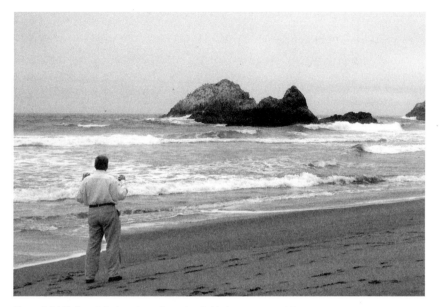

Figure 1.5. We forget that we have the potential to improve our vision.

I've proven the conventional wisdom wrong and have shown the power of healing exercises.

I am grateful that Miriam and Jacob taught me eye exercises and body movement, and encouraged me to share these exercises with other people. I have met people who have improved their bodies even from major conditions such as paralysis from polio, motor neuron disease, muscular dystrophy, spinal injuries, arthritis, strokes, and many other ailments. I knew I had found my calling: to bring this consciousness to others. Most people have little faith in their own healing ability. My faith in their ability is great because of my faith in my own ability and my success.

There are two ways for me to describe to you how you can improve. One is to explain that the body has a greater functional potential than most people ever experience in life. The other is to demonstrate how to meet that potential through exercise. Whenever I work with people, I demonstrate to them that they can do more than they think. When they have pain, this means helping them not let the pain restrict them too much. When they have tension, it means first helping them recognize the tension to its fullest extent, then decreasing it.

My own process was not smooth. My eyes used to involuntarily move three hundred times per minute until I learned to palm: rubbing my hands, putting them around my eye orbits very gently, and visualizing darkness. This would calm and relax my eyes. In one strange way, it actually helped to have deaf parents in my teens. I could play loud rock and roll music and relax with it. In spite of our thin walls, my parents couldn't hear it. Whenever I played this music, I would place my hands very gently around my eye orbits to relax my eyes. The movement of my eyes decreased to sixty movements per minute within three months. That's when my vision started to clear. The exercise of sunning warmed my eyes and started to activate my irregular pupils.

Although I could not exactly see, I gradually learned to look, even though it was sometimes painful. I had been taught by my Braille teacher to "feel the Braille and not look at the page. For God's sake, don't look, because if you look, you'll confuse your senses. You've got to *feel* and not *look*." That order was so vigorous that I had learned to live a life without

Figure 1.6. My eyes used to move involuntarily three hundred times per minute until I learned palming.

looking at anything. Looking was a new order to my brain. The result, even though I was starting to see more, was that my eyes hurt. Palming and lying down for a long time had helped me. Sometimes I just didn't want to see anything; it was just too much. But I kept looking.

When I arrived in the United States, I met some people who were very interested in my work. They offered to help me train other people in my methods. It was new to me to have people embrace my experiences. I learned how to teach individuals—as Miriam always taught me only to work with individuals—and how to teach classes in a way that would enable each individual to learn how to work with himself or herself. From this I learned that the greatest difficulty most people have is that they don't believe they can find the time to work on themselves. Most people think they are too busy. Others feel impatient and aren't willing to invest the effort it takes to quiet and to relax their minds and bodies. I teach them how to incorporate these exercises into their existing routines. I teach them that looking at details is something they had stopped being motivated to do a long time ago, and to do so stimulates the macula and can prevent macular degeneration. I teach them that sitting with a loose neck is worth the investment of moving the head in a rotating motion before sitting in a chair. I teach people that, while they use their computers, they should look far away from time to time to rest their eyes. These are simple habits that are easily incorporated into day-to-day life.

My own two children were born with cataracts, which was traumatic for me and for their mother, as we knew from experience the struggle they would face. At the age of two weeks, they went through cataract surgeries that allowed the visual brain to develop normally. This was unknown in my generation. Because their surgeries were successful, they did not have to deal with the scarring that I dealt with when I was young. Using the techniques you will read about in this book, their vision has improved tremendously. Throughout their childhood and adolescence, my children have sat in my car, covering their strong eyes, and looking with their weak eyes at objects, in order to ease the strain of looking with the strong eyes all the time.

With an artist's mind and an artist's heart, my son, Gull, is often in his own world in many ways. While in his world, however, he looks at details with great interest. Because of his powerful capacity of observation and love of detail, he sees much that others don't see. It is an amazing inside world that relates to both his artistic mind and his autism. While I feel that his surgery was very successful, it's possible that the combination of treatments—some electric treatments, and also anesthesia—have, to some extent, affected his brain. Yet, his internal world is amazing. Unfortunately, many people don't see it because he's afflicted with a very mild form of autism. But anyone who does acknowledge that world sees an amazing person with a kind heart and deep perception. In fact, he has the ability to discern details that most people tend to ignore most of their lives.

Gull has developed the best vision of any kid who was ever born with cataracts. He now sees at 20/40 without glasses. This is 80 percent of 20/20 vision, without his natural lenses. Anyone else without the natural lens of the eye would be seeing 20/400 (5 percent of normal vision). He sees 20/15 with glasses. Most other kids who were born with cataracts and had successful surgeries see 20/80 or 20/100 using much thicker lenses; 20/40 is unheard-of vision for someone who has no natural lens of his own.

My daughter has also passed through many transitions. We used to play a lot of games in our living room, where she would cover her strong eye and play ball with me using her weaker eye. Seeing that ball as it rolled close and far made a huge difference for her, and her vision greatly improved. At the age of twelve, she developed elevated eye pressure. Immediately, the doctors wanted to give her eyedrops to reduce her pressure. We declined the doctors' recommendation because we believed the drops could be damaging. I worked with her instead and, in spite of incredibly demanding middle school and high school schedules with many extracurricular activities, she found some time to work on her periphery, which reduced the eye pressure. She also found some time to work on her neck. She saw acupuncturists, took homeopathy diligently, took vitamin treatments, and got massage treatments to reduce the tension in her back and neck. I taught her how to relax her whole body in many different ways in order to bring more blood circulation to her head. Her pressure was reduced enormously. And to this day she has not taken eyedrops.

The process was long, hard, and cumbersome, and had its ups and downs, but it worked. With high pressure, some people have a tendency toward developing glaucoma, and glaucoma expresses itself by damaging the optic nerve and diminishing the field of vision. So our success with her is partial but good; her vision is 20/20. Though her tendency is for high pressure, her optic nerve is very healthy and her field of vision is excellent.

From these experiences of my own, with my children, and with thousands of patients and students with whom I've worked, I have come to truly believe that people can improve their vision and find the time to do so, whether they're in school or in the workplace.

A wonderful computer engineer who once came to a class of mine was able to improve his vision from 20/200 to 20/80 during the class. He reduced his prescription by half within eight months, from 7 diopters to 3.5 diopters. For the first time in his adult life, and still in his forties, he felt comfortable driving in the daytime without glasses.

We all can take the time. We just have to decide that we are worth the time, and that the process is worth our while. We need to make an effort to combine eye exercises with our everyday lives. Then we can thrive. Then we can excel. Imagine never needing to have any major treatments from the eye doctor. Imagine your life without cataracts, macular degeneration, glaucoma, or retinal detachment. Imagine that you can improve your life simply by creating more life in your eyes.

So far, the oldest person I've worked with was 101 years old. This patient experienced great changes and was able to see better and to improve his brain and eye functions quite a bit, even after one session. Since he was one of only two patients over the age of 100 with whom I've worked, I can only give these examples. I did, however, have success with both of them. I have also worked with several patients in their eighties and nineties, and have witnessed tremendous positive changes in their visual systems through working with these exercises.

There is no doubt in my mind that, whether you are in your twenties, thirties, forties, fifties, sixties, or seventies, you can change the function of your eyes. There is enough elasticity in your brain to back it up. The problem isn't age itself, but whether or not a person is practicing the correct exercises for his or her age. It may be easier for a five-year-old child to get used to the weaker eye's workings by putting on a patch for four or eight hours a day as he or she plays. And truly, the brain has more plasticity when you're five than when you're seventy-five. But there are good age-appropriate exercises you can do at any time in your life that can change your visual system completely.

Chapter 2

Ten Steps to Better Vision

If you take care of your vision, not only will you see better, you will also feel better, and you will positively affect your whole body's health. In addition to the exercises aimed at combating specific disorders and conditions, I have developed ten important exercises that are perfect for incorporating into your daily life. These exercises are based on my nine principles of healthy vision:

1. Deep Relaxation
2. Adjusting to Light Frequencies
3. Looking at Details
4. Looking into the Distance
5. Expanding Your Periphery
6. Balanced Use of the Two Eyes
7. Balanced Use within Each Eye
8. Body and Eye Coordination
9. Having Adequate Blood Flow to Nourish the Eyes
10. Vision and Body

These are the essential principles of healthy vision, and can be attained by consistently practicing the nine fundamental eye exercises in this chapter.

Step 1: The Long Swing

I will never forget when I met Alan. He was a young French-Canadian banker who, while driving home after a long and tiring meeting at his bank, fell asleep at the wheel and found himself in intensive care three days later. By the time he woke up, they had replaced his forehead with platinum. He had lost all his vision. The optic nerve in his left eye was destroyed, in addition to most of the optic nerve in his right eye. But that little bit of nerve tissue remained, so Alan discovered that he still had some visual sensation.

The physicians thought that only four percent of his potentially functional nerve was not enough to regain any vision. Alan heard about my book *The Handbook of Self-Healing*. In it, I suggested that people who are legally blind start working with blinking lights in a dark room. Alan experimented with the techniques in the book, and sure enough, the little bit of remaining optic nerve woke up. He called me in San Francisco and soon came out for a series of therapy sessions. Alan's girlfriend held his hand to walk him into the office because he couldn't see most objects. His brain did not yet know how to use that little bit of remaining healthy nerve tissue in his right eye.

During our first session, we practiced an exercise called *the long swing*. As he did this exercise, he said, "I'm noticing twelve objects that I've never noticed before in the room." Within minutes, his sense of orientation built up even more. When the series of sessions finished, he no longer needed to be led around. The long swing is what is called an integrative exercise. It allowed Alan to perceive a sense of space.

The long swing exercise develops a sense of fluidity and flexibility that will allow you to look at details with more ease, to adapt to light more easily, and to adapt to new, livelier visual habits.

How to Do the Long Swing

Stand with your legs slightly more than hip width apart, and your knees slightly bent. Hold your index finger about one foot in front of your face, pointing up to the ceiling. Look at your finger with a soft gaze. If you are legally blind, or even with correction have very poor vision, you can look at your index and middle fingers together. While looking at your finger, swing your body from side to side. As you swing to the right, twist your body so that your left heel rises slightly off the ground. As you twist your body to the left, your right heel raises slightly off the ground. If your hand becomes tired, you can switch hands. Do this at least twenty times.

You will notice the sensation that everything in the background seems to be moving in the opposite direction of your finger, like scenery passing by you as you look out the window of a train. Allow yourself to feel the sense of relaxation that comes when you don't need to place a hard focus on any one object. Move to the right, and the world moves to the left.

Move the left, and the world moves to the right. Move slowly, and the world will move fast for you.

Figure 2.1. Long swing, front view (a). Keep your eye on your finger. Long swing, right profile (b). Long swing, left profile (c).

Now hold your finger horizontally in front of your face. Move your finger up and down in front of you, moving your head vertically along with your finger. Remember to continue to hold a soft gaze. When you move up, everything in the background seems to be moving down. When you move down, everything seems to be moving up.

Next, hold your finger in front of you and do the long swing, pointing your finger to the ceiling as in the first explanation, but this time, as you swing to one side, bend at the waist and sweep down in a half circle—just to knee level. Don't lower your head below your knees, but continue the swing until your arm is fully extended and you are looking up at your finger. This exercise should relax your eyes further.

The next step is very important. This is where we visualize the long swing. We close our eyes and do the movement with our bodies, and visualize in our mind's eye that the world is swinging back and forth, passing in front of our eyes. Everything you visualize is moving directly opposite. When you move to the right, the neighborhood moves to the left. When you move to the left, the neighborhood moves to the right. Remember how you saw objects this way. Now visualize the whole world moving in the opposite direction of your swing. Now you open your eyes and continue the exercise.

When you look in this way, you stop yourself from freezing. It becomes easier to look at details and much easier to blink. Remind yourself to blink. Blinking will help you to relax.

When I started to work on my own vision, my eyes had a constant nystagmus, which is an involuntary rapid movement of the eyes caused by continuous strain from trying and see the world with a total lack of success. So I practiced the long swing for about forty minutes a day, and it immediately eased the involuntary flutter of my eyes. I had a feeling of more light entering my eyes. Details started to appear in the background, and when I started to look at details like windows and books on shelves, they gradually became clearer and clearer to me. Long swinging prepared my brain for new exercises.

When you practice the rest of the exercises in this book followed by long swinging, you will absorb the exercises better because long swinging alleviates tension and stiffness in the brain, in addition to preparing us to learn and benefit from new visual techniques.

I will never forget the time when I was walking in the streets of Tel Aviv with my eye instructor, Jacob, who was then only sixteen years old. Jacob told me to look at a building full of windows. In the corner of the windows I could see tiny, fuzzy black squares, which I later realized were air conditioners. At Jacob's instruction, I looked from window to air conditioner, back and forth for a whole summer, not understanding why I was doing this. Slowly, by looking at windows and air conditioners, looking at patterns of squares, a new habit developed in me: a habit of looking and not freezing. Long swinging helped to prepare me for this exercise and alleviated the rigidity that prevented me from looking at details, which allowed the program to sink in.

The reason that long swinging is referred to as an integrative exercise is that it takes you away from the stress you're used to. When people wear thick glasses that have a very specific focal point, they often strain their eyes so much that it becomes very difficult for them to look with vitality at the world. They look without seeing details, partially from fatigue and partially from the habits they have developed by straining to see. Long swinging breaks that tension. You cannot stare with this exercise, so more light enters your eyes through the movement; therefore you won't need to strain to bring the new programming to your brain.

The long swinging exercise will also help you develop your peripheral vision and create a better sense of orientation. You don't have to swing for forty minutes at a time. In fact, even two minutes of twenty swings can help you loosen up. Think of it as warming up before a workout.

Step 2: Looking into the Distance

It is no coincidence that our school is located near the beach. In fact, it took us almost five years to convince San Francisco authorities and neighborhood groups to allow us to operate in this residential area. The reason this location is ideal for us is that we look at the waves on a daily basis and use their sparkling beauty in our work. They shine in sunlight and have different coloration, even in the fog. You can almost always see waves here, even when the weather is gray.

Look at the waves. Look at the sky. Look at the clouds. Look at the hills and valleys. If you are not near the beach, look out your window at the many other buildings.

When you look near, as when staring at a computer screen, you unknowingly strain your eyes. The ciliary muscles contract, and this changes the shape of your lens from flat to round. When you look into the distance, however, the ciliary muscles relax and the suspensory ligaments keep the lens flat, and more flexible.

Many people in our culture are used to eyestrain from looking at computers, televisions, and books so much of the time. They pay attention to the contents and not to their eyes, which causes them to strain. Looking close makes you strain. Looking with boredom makes you strain. When you strain your eyes—even when you are aware of the strain—you push on with the computer project, or the television show, or the book.

Pay attention so that your face is relaxed and your jaw is not clenched. Release and rest your eyes. If it is possible, give yourself a few hours away

Figure 2.2. The reason this location is ideal for us is that we look at the waves on a daily basis and use their sparkling beauty in our work.

from close work. Even if it is a deadline you are struggling to meet, do yourself a favor and take ten minutes to rest your eyes by looking into the distance. Look at the movements of the waves or the clouds. *Look into the distance.*

Never look closer than forty yards away, because you need to look far enough to rest the eyes from looking near. Know that when you look into the distance, you don't have to stay focused on one point; in a soft way, you can scan or look from point to point at various details of what you see in the distance or the horizon. Remember to blink and never strain to see the distance or the horizon. If it is fuzzy, let it be fuzzy. From time to time, rapidly wave your hands to the side of your face, without looking at your hands, just noticing them or their movement. Do not do this all the time. Sometimes, massage your face from the bridge of the nose to the temples over the eyebrows on the frontal bone. Massage below your eyes from the nose to the ears, over the cheekbone, while looking into the distance. Waving your hands to the side quickly will help you adjust to the light more easily by expanding the areas of the retina that absorb it, and create balance.

DISCOVERING YOUR STRONG EYE

About 20 percent of the people that I've met have no difference in strength between their two eyes. Even so, the majority of people do have very different levels of strength between their eyes. A small number of those people have one eye stronger for looking from a distance, and the other is stronger for looking from nearby.

If you experience an extreme difference of ability between your two eyes, you probably already know it by now. You may know which eye needs a stronger prescription for correction. You may have had an injury to one of your eyes, or you may simply be aware of which eye you mainly use to look. If you are not sure which one of your eyes is your dominant eye, there is a way you can test it.

To see which eye is dominant for distance, make a loose fist with a pencil-sized hole through the center, like a telescope. Hold your loose fist about a foot away from your face. It can be closer for people who see poorly or farther for people who see sharply, as long as it is far enough away that you are looking with both eyes at the same time. Look at some distant point through the hole in your fist. Now close one eye and see if that point disappears. For example, if your stronger eye is your left eye, when you close the right eye, you will still see the object through your fist. When you close the left eye, you will not see the object, and vice versa. Then you'll know which eye of yours is stronger. At times this stronger eye will be the only eye working. This can be taxing on that eye and debilitate the weaker eye from lack of use, and you won't even know this is happening.

To see which eye is dominant for near, look at the pages in this book with the large and small print. Look at the smallest letters you can see, then close one eye at a time. Whichever eye can see the small letters better is your strong eye for nearby vision.

If you cannot figure out on your own which eye is stronger, you can go to an optometrist and ask for help.

Figure 2.3. Discovering the dominant eye.

Look into the distance for at least twenty minutes a day. If you wear corrective lenses, be brave: take your contact lenses out, take your glasses off, and allow your eyes to enjoy a breath of fresh air. One student in San Francisco came to me and said that after two and a half weeks of not wearing her lenses, she had started to feel comfortable, because of "the air bouncing on her eyes." This habit will reduce your dependency on glasses or lenses, and it will gradually strengthen your visual system.

And while I prefer that you look into the distance eight to ten minutes three times a day, it may not be part of your reality. The minimum that anyone should do this exercise is in intervals of four to six minutes. So if you did it twenty minutes a day in four- to six-minute intervals, four times a day, it may end up preventing cataracts, and it will also relax your eyes.

Looking into the Distance Can Help Prevent Cataracts

If you can share this simple concept with other people, you will help to create a revolution in the world by helping to prevent the predictable cataract. Today, most physicians believe that, sooner or later, most people will develop cataracts. Looking into the distance can prevent the onset of cataracts because it gives the lens its full mobility and more life.

I admit that even if you practice this exercise every day, you will probably not look into the distance as much as life requires you to look near. Nevertheless, looking into the distance for eight to ten minutes, three times a day, will at least allow your eyes to rest, and will compensate for the strain of looking near.

Step 3: Exploring the Periphery

It is impossible to strain your eyes while looking centrally if you remember to simultaneously focus on your periphery. In our culture, we suppress parts of the eye that help us to see well naturally. It is a subconscious suppression. The reason we suppress the periphery is because we make it irrelevant to our lives. As we focus on objects in front of us, we simply don't pay attention to what's around us. On the other hand, our ancient fathers and mothers, our predecessors, had to pay attention to it; in the jungle, you wouldn't last more than a week without noticing the periphery. In fact, you would be eaten or you would starve to death if you don't notice what was around you.

But we ignore the periphery so we can focus on computers and paperwork all day without being distracted by our environment. We try to concentrate on the task at hand, not to be distracted by the commotion around us. When we don't notice the periphery, the strain on our central vision becomes much greater, which in time makes us use it poorly. This causes us to strain our central vision, decreasing its clarity and eventually losing it. The old adage that says "use it or lose it" holds true here. With time, we lose the connection between our brain, our optic nerve, and the rod cells of the periphery. Along with genetic tendencies, this can be a cause of glaucoma.

What we need to do right now is to exercise our periphery. You will feel that there is integration of the periphery and the center, and as a result you'll have a sense of more brightness and more light in your eyes.

Periphery Exercise 1: Look into the Distance

Sit somewhere comfortable where you can see something in the distance that you enjoy looking at. As you look into the distance, start to wave your hands quickly to the side of your head to notify your eyes that a periphery exists. Don't look at your hands waving, Just look into the distance. Allow your eyes to recognize the movement of your hands. Wave your hands quickly in such a way that your fingers point toward you and your wrists are loose. Do this for a minute or two. As you do this, you should feel your eyes release their tension; this relaxation in your eyes is vitally important to healthy vision.

Figure 2.4. Will wakes up his periphery with a wave of his hands as he looks at the distance.

Periphery Exercise 2: Small Pieces of Paper

Cut out a small piece of opaque paper, about one and a half inches by two inches, and tape the paper horizontally on the bridge of your nose, so that it is centered between your eyes. This will disrupt part of your central vision.

Walk around in a familiar environment with this paper on your nose for a minute or two. Now sit down and wave your hands quickly to the side of your head like you did before. Then, rock forward toward your

thighs and back up again, bending at the hips, while you wave your hands to the side quickly. Stand up and sit down several times, moving your whole body up and down, as you wave your hands quickly to the side. As you do this, it reveals to your brain the existence of a moving periphery with which it normally does not connect.

Figure 2.5. Will uses the smallest piece of paper to block his central vision while activating his periphery.

In the past, people used to walk at night, sometimes in total darkness and sometimes with light from the stars and the moon. Imagine how important it was for them to notice things moving in their periphery at night! For millions of years, our ancestors used to walk this way. Now we have the city lights at night, and our peripheral cells are hardly being used, because they are mainly designed for night vision.

Waving our hands to our sides wakes up the peripheral cells because the rods of the retina respond to movement rather than to still images; conversely, the cones respond better to a still picture. These cones are mainly in the central part of the retina—the area called the macula—and are used to look at details. An overwhelming number of the retina's cells are the rods, which respond mostly to the impression of movement. When we exercise these rods, we take away a lot of stress from the overworked cones, and we make it easier for them to function more correctly. Instead of the brain forcing the eye to freeze and strenuously see a picture, the

Figure 2.6. Will blocks even more of his central vision (a). As he waves, he leans forward and back in a rocking motion to create more movement in his periphery (b).

brain will command the eye to look gently and easily in order to see the entire landscape better.

Next, put a longer piece of paper, one inch by five inches, on the bridge of your nose, and repeat this exercise. Then, use a paper that is one inch by seven inches. By blocking so much of your central vision, and even some of your peripheral vision, you will discover a periphery that you hardly ever use consciously. Now go back to the medium-size paper and repeat the exercise. Then use the small piece of paper and repeat the exercise a final time. You may find that a small paper now seems even smaller in your perception. That is because much of your brain that had been suppressed is now engaged in peripheral vision.

To finish, take the small paper off, stand, and do the long swing so your brain will absorb the exercise you have just performed.

Step 4: Sunning and Skying

Surrendering to the sun briefly each day can make a huge difference in terms of our overall feeling of well-being.

Since the 1980s, physicians have warned us against the dangers of exposure to the sun. Now they understand the benefits of sunlight, and recommend that we have some exposure to it daily. The sun is one of the best nurturers that nature has given us. It is important, however, to adapt your eyes to the strong light of the sun. Sunning is a great exercise for this purpose because it is relaxing to the eyes and it can also help you with your sleep.

I once had a patient who complained about terrible insomnia. She had not slept for many nights and had a tremendous amount of tension. I taught her the sunning exercise, and massaged her in the sun. After her first session, she went home and slept right through the night; after taking only three sessions at the clinic of the school, she reported that she had slept much better. That was years ago. To this day, she practices the sunning technique and has no more sleep deprivation.

Today, physicians suggest that we should not expose ourselves to the sun, except before 10 a.m. and after 5 p.m. In my opinion, we should sometimes expose ourselves to the sun even at midday. If you are sensitive to sunlight, you should start by practicing the sunning exercise early in the morning or near dusk, or for just five minutes at a time in the middle of the day.

To begin sunning, all you need to do is close your eyes and face the sun. Now move your head from side to side, rotating it from shoulder to shoulder. As you face the sun, the iris sphincter muscles constrict the pupils. As you move your head away toward one shoulder, the radial dilator muscles dilate the pupils, even though your eyes are closed. For some people, it is easy to move their head 180 degrees from shoulder to shoulder. If you find this full range of motion difficult, simply bring your opposite shoulder forward slightly; it will help you move your head all the way toward the side, and compensate for the limited range of motion until you loosen up. The more you practice this exercise, the more your range of motion and flexibility will increase.

The movements should not be fast, but they should not be slow either. Just relax, breathe deeply and slowly, and visualize that the sun, with its energy and light, is penetrating your face and nurturing your eyes as well as your mind. Your eyelids should be closed softly; don't squeeze your eyelids shut. You want the eyelids to close as gently as if you were about to go to sleep. The less you squeeze your eyelids, the more relaxed your eyes will become.

When I was in high school, I was doing this sunning exercise on a camping trip. Seeing me rotate my head back and forth, a girl asked,

Figure 2.7. Move your head from side to side, rotating it from shoulder to shoulder (a). As you face the sun, the iris sphincter muscles constrict the pupils even with your eyes closed (b). Move your opposite shoulder slightly forward if your neck does not move as freely as this yoga student's (c).

"Why do you keep saying no? Can't you say yes?" So I moved my head up and down as if to nod "yes," and I had a revelation. I noticed that this movement led to a greater variability in the angles at which light reached my eyes, thus awakening more parts of them. This additional exercise allowed for greater stimulation and increased sensation of lightness and darkness. I recommend this additional exercise be included during sunning.

Whenever you experience that difference between extremes of dark and light, your pupils become stronger. The pupils of most modern people are very weak because they wear sunglasses when they're outside, which weakens the pupils. Automatic activities, like those of the eye's iris muscles that affect the pupils, are influenced by function and use. The more you constrict and expand your pupils, the stronger the iris muscles become. Your retina also benefits from more concentrated light, and blood flows much better to the eye as a result of the pupils contracting and expanding. There are several additional benefits. One is that it wakes up your macula and reinforces its function, which is the most important part of the retina for clear central vision. Two, it boosts your optimism when sunlight meets the red blood cells: it stimulates their activity, especially of the hemoglobin in them, which leads to secretion of serotonin from the brain, which creates a good mood more effectively than any drug. Three, it boosts your immune system. It also helps boost vitamin D, which helps your bones and muscle contraction and improves blood flow.

The sunning exercise is mandatory for people who want to improve their vision. Like any exercise, it doesn't create drastic change for everyone. But quite a few of my clients have experienced huge vision improvement and have reduced the strength of their eyeglasses prescriptions when they have diligently practiced sunning. When you have a break at work or school, I recommend sunning instead of smoking cigarettes or drinking coffee.

Skying

Skying is a simple exercise. It is similar to sunning, but you do this when there is no sun. You just put one hand behind the back of your head and one hand on your forehead, applying pressure so that you massage your head as you turn it from side to side. Now move your head from side to side like you are sunning and blink rapidly at the sky.

After two minutes of skying, do one minute of the long swing. Stand with your legs slightly more than hip width apart, and your knees slightly bent. Hold your index finger about one foot in front of your face, pointing up to the ceiling. Look at your finger with a soft gaze. While looking at your finger, swing your body from side to side. As you swing to the right, twist your body so that your left heel rises slightly off the ground. As you twist your body to the left, your right heel raises slightly off the ground. Then do three minutes of skying and two minutes of swinging. Then do three more minutes of skying and two more minutes of swinging. This is an anti-squinting exercise and, as you sky and then swing, you are letting

Figure 2.8. Apply great pressure to the head, holding the arms raised as you blink at the sky and turn only your head from side to side. Long swinging and skying go hand in hand.

more light into your eyes and stopping the tendency to squint. You may find that the light bothers you less after doing the long swing.

Step 5: Night Walking

A complementary exercise to sunning is called night walking. The idea is simply to walk at night, in the dark, with only the light of the moon and the stars to guide your way.

Most of us, even if we live outside a city, are surrounded by the glow of city lights. Those of us who live in remote areas often use flashlights. We have all learned to live with artificial lights, but once you get completely away from them for a time, you begin to realize how profoundly the city lights burden your eyes. Yes, we are happy to have them because they light the streets, making us safer and allowing for activity after the sun has set. But remember, as valuable as they may be to our industry and safety, this constant light is not beneficial to our eyes. For this reason, we must take part in exercises like night walking that strengthen our eyes and compensate for the burden of city lights.

Every time I teach an extensive eye course, we spend one evening in which we walk together in the dark. It is very pleasant for all of us to walk in places like the park, where we are free from artificial light. Of course, it can be dangerous to walk in the dark, whether you live in the city or in the country, so I recommend that, when practicing night walking, you get a group of friends to walk together.

In the dark of night, it only takes three to four minutes to expand your pupils to nine times the size they normally contract to in the daytime. It takes about forty minutes to wake up the rods of the retina that sense movement and periphery. After night walking for about fifty minutes, you are finally utilizing all of your eyes' potential.

Night walking is a wonderful opportunity to try all the other exercises you are learning. After finding a nice, safe place to walk in the dark, set out and explore the many benefits of this practice. During your walk, stop at times and do the long swing exercise. Allow yourself the time to adjust to the darkness, and let your brain comprehend the change it is experiencing.

Short palming for fifteen to forty-five seconds is another exercise that works great as an addition to night walking because it allows your eyes to better adjust to the dark. After they have properly adjusted, you can try peripheral exercises if you feel secure in your surroundings. Tape a short piece of paper between your eyes, and wave your hands quickly to the sides of your head while walking to wake up the periphery.

By the time you finish your night walking, you will have awakened your eyes and reminded your brain of the way it used to function in a more primitive time, before light pollution filled the earth. Therefore, if you are serious about improving your eyes, night walking is an effective and enjoyable exercise that I would recommend doing at least twice a month when weather permits.

Step 6: Palming

Caution: Before palming, glaucoma patients should look at the section on glaucoma in chapter 6 for important modifications to this exercise.

This exercise is one that Tibetan yogis have been practicing for more than 1,500 years. It is an exercise that complements every other practice you will learn from this book, and it is called palming.

Many people believe that they receive sufficient rest for their eyes while they are asleep. While sleep is very important, even with adequate sleep, many people still experience eye fatigue. There are a few reasons why this happens. One reason is that, in these modern times, we often hear noise around us while we are asleep; even though we don't feel disturbed, the noise upsets our rest on a subconscious level. The other reason sleep often fails to sufficiently rest our eyes is that many people sleep in rooms that are not completely dark. I suggest that you darken your bedroom all you can. The darker the room, the more rest you will give your eyes. Sleeping in total darkness produces hormones, like melatonin, that relax your body, allowing you to experience deeper and more refreshing sleep.

In order for sleep to be completely satisfying, quite often we dream. Dreams enhance our state of being; it is as though they wash away the day. Although dreams allow for physical and mental relaxation, the saccadic movement during dreams doesn't allow for full relaxation of the eyes.

The greatest rest is conscious rest, not passive rest. William Bates, the originator of eye exercises in the modern world, understood this principle. And the Tibetan yogis, who have mastered the art of meditation, understand this concept perhaps even better than anyone else. When you meditate, you enter a state of transcendent relaxation. Like with meditation, palming helps us to quiet the mind and focus on eye relaxation. This produces a very powerful effect. There is a great Jewish adage that says "the truth is always simple." The way to the truth, however, may be complex and full of obstacles.

To palm correctly, and to receive the benefits of this powerful exercise, you first have to engage in the correct preparation. You must have relaxed hands because this exercise takes you to a place where your hands nurture your eyes. Healthy hands can bring warmth, energy, and blood flow to the eyes, but there is no way for you to energize your eyes if your hands are angry, irritated, or numb in any way. The cells of the hands will communicate relaxation to the cells of the eyes. More and more people understand that there is cell communication. This exercise depends on good communication between loving hands and eyes that need nurturing and relaxation. Ensuring relaxed hands is necessary to receive benefits from this exercise.

Preparing to Palm

The most important thing when palming is that you are not stressed. I recommend massaging your temples, face, shoulders, and the top of your head in order to bring good blood flow to the eyes and become as relaxed as possible.

Loosen your shoulders. Move your shoulders together in a rotating motion, forward and then back. Then rotate each shoulder separately, forward and back. Picture that the shoulder tip is moving the shoulder. Now tap on the tip of the shoulder with your opposite hand and say out loud, "shoulder tip." Moving the shoulders in a rotating motion increases blood circulation; as you repeat this exercise several times, your shoulders will feel lighter.

Next, lift your arm up and move your whole arm in a rotating motion, imagining that your fingertips are moving your arm. By focusing on your

Figure 2.9. Massage the scalp and temple (a). Massage the cheek bones (b). Massage the scalp (c). Massage the neck (d).

fingertips, your body will naturally loosen. Tap the wall or your thigh with your fingertips and say, "fingertips." Then put your opposite hand on your shoulder and move it in a rotating motion. After tapping on the tip of your shoulders and then tapping with your fingertips on the wall, tap on your shoulder and the wall at the same time and then move your arm in rotating motion, thinking that the fingertips are moving the arm; and then move the shoulder in rotating motion, thinking that the tip of the shoulder is moving the shoulder. While it is not anatomically correct that the shoulder or the fingertips are making the movement, thinking this way helps you use the proper muscles, which leads to a great loosening effect and not tensing the muscles that do not belong to that motion. Repeat this series of movements with the opposite shoulder and hand.

Figure 2.10. Move your shoulders together in a rotating motion, forward and then back (a). Intertwine your fingers, straighten your arms, and move your arms in a circular motion (b).

Quite often the area between the shoulders gets contracted and, in a way, energy becomes trapped because there is not enough movement happening in that area. Consequently, there is not enough blood flow, which quite literally freezes the hands.

The next step for palming is to open and close your fingers one hundred times, visualizing that the fingertips are initiating the movement. From time to time, tap with your fingertips on the opposite forearm. Now massage your hands, front and back, by pretending you are washing them with soap and water. Make sure that your elbows are placed at an elevation just below the shoulders; you can use a few pillows on a table, or a palming stick, which is an adjustable rod that can move up and down, with a platform on top on which you can rest your elbows. The neck remains straight. Don't wrench your neck, don't tilt your head forward or back, but remain straight. Some people lie down when they do palming. They put two pillows behind their head, and three pillows between the elbows and the knees. The two things that are not allowed when you are palming are elevating your shoulders and putting pressure on your cheekbones. Once comfortably positioned, briskly rub your palms together, as though you are trying to warm them.

Figure 2.11. Rub your palms together to warm them (a). Place the palms very gently over the eye orbits, putting no pressure on the face (b).

The result of this exercise is that your fingers will be warm and your hands will be loose. The warmth and relaxation of your hands will enable you now to palm in a way that is correct and beneficial. Though it is very important to be relaxed while palming, not all of these shoulder exercises will always be necessary. At the very least, rub your palms together to warm them; then intertwine your fingers, straighten your arms, and move your arms in a circular motion. Utilize your full range of motion several times in both directions, first with your hands palm to palm, and then with your palms facing outward. Depending on the time available, these relaxation exercises may last anywhere between two and eight minutes.

How to Palm

Now that you have prepared your body for palming, sit somewhere comfortable. You need to have your elbows resting on pillows or on a tabletop with a pillow so that your head is leaning neither forward nor backward. In other words, you are sitting comfortably in good posture. It is very important that you are not holding your arms up, that you are not straining your neck by letting your head tilt back, and most important, that you never put any pressure on your face at all. If you put your weight on anything, it is on your elbows.

Rub your palms together to warm them and place them very gently over the eye orbits. The palms never touch the eyelids, but notice how your palms feel *over* your eyelids, over the entire eye orbit. Can you feel the warmth? Do your hands feel nurturing as they sit ever so lightly over your eye orbits? This is important. If you are stressed or angry, your palming session will not feel good. Repeat the exercises to prepare for palming or do some kind of activity that helps you to let go of the stress or the anger you are carrying.

Visualization While Palming

While you palm, there are two visualizations that will help you to receive the full benefit of this exercise. The first is that you visualize a figure eight, or an infinity symbol. You can visualize a boat on the ocean moving in the figure-eight pattern, or a train in the mountains traveling a route shaped like the infinity symbol. This is a fluid movement that helps your mind be able to travel from detail to detail easily and fluidly.

The second visualization is of total blackness and increasing blackness. Close your eyes and begin palming. Now visualize that the room you are in is being painted black. Visualize that your body is being painted black. Visualize that the neighborhood is being painted black. Visualize that the city is being painted black. Visualize black paint covering the entire world. Visualize that all the stars and the sun are being painted black. This is total blackness you are visualizing. Black is the color that allows the optic nerve to relax.

Breathing While Palming

Remember to inhale and exhale slowly while palming. Visualize your abdomen rising slowly and falling gently. Count to eight as you slowly breathe in, then count to eleven as you slowly breathe out. Inhalation is slow. Exhalation is slower. Don't tense up; just let yourself breathe in and out through your nose.

Right now, you feel that your whole upper torso is expanding while you inhale, and shrinking as you exhale. At the same time, you should feel that your head expands as you inhale and shrinks as you exhale. You visualize that your pelvis expands as you inhale and shrinks as you exhale, or that your legs expand as you breathe in and shrink as you breathe out. You visualize that your whole body expands as you breathe in and shrinks as you breathe out.

Often your hearing becomes more acute while palming. After you've finished palming, it's good to put your thumbs in your ears, breathe deeply, and listen to the breath. It sounds like ocean waves or wind. Your thumbs should be deep, but not forced.

Relaxing the Ears

A good addition to palming the eyes is resting the ears from external noise. As a result of the noise we live in, our senses are under continuous pressure. Pressure causes tension, and if we are tense, we can never get to a place of relaxed eyes.

So, when you finish palming, rub your hands together again to increase the blood flow to your fingers, then put your thumbs deep inside your ears. Listen to your breath. What does it sound like? It may sound like ocean waves or wind. Breathe deeply and slowly and count to ten, and palm again. You will feel your neck muscles becoming loose, and your whole head will start to relax.

Figure 2.12. Put your thumbs deep inside your ears. Listen to your breath.

How Long Should You Palm?

The duration of your palming may change depending on your schedule and your state of mind. If you are busy, perhaps you might take a break in the middle of your work from time to time, and sit for a few minutes to palm. You can palm for one minute just to rest the eyes, but it takes a minimum of six minutes to clear the retina from neurological waste products. Of course, it is even more wonderful if you can palm for fifteen or twenty minutes at a time.

Benefits of Palming

People who have multiple sclerosis and have an attack on their visual system quite often receive cortisone treatments or other steroids from their doctors. In many cases, if such patients just sat down for a whole day palming with a nice cloth around their eyes, they would be able to overcome the attack on the visual system simply through rest. It's a simple truth that relaxation is very powerful. When you relax completely, your body returns to its highest and best functioning.

I am in awe of nature for giving us such wonderful tools with which to see. In all its complexity, nature has fine-tuned our vision. Vision is completely integrated with our development as human beings, and is progressing side by side with it. Most of the visual process is subconscious and unknown to us. But science is gradually realizing the marvelous energy behind vision.

We have 126 million photoreceptor cells in each retina, with a billion light rays bouncing against some of them every single minute, converting light into visual energy. To allow the process to function at its best, we need to learn not to squint. You may not be aware that your eyes squint even when you sleep and dream.

Palming can work away our tendency to squint. When you palm with soft, relaxed hands, and when you see black, there is a wonderful release of the eyelids, the temples, the forehead, and the entire skull. Squinting is eliminated, and you notice a relaxed sensation as you open your eyes. You also sense much more periphery because, with fully open eyelids, much more light can penetrate your eyes.

Quite often, physicians say that squinting does not have any ill effects, but it does. In this respect, the wisdom of the Tibetan yogis was definitely greater than the wisdom of modern medicine. Modern medicine still needs to adopt the concept that rest and relaxation are powerful.

Combining Palming with Other Exercises

After you have mastered palming, next time you are sunning, or practicing the long swing or night walking, stop for a few moments, put your hands over your eye orbits, and do your palming. It takes a minimum of six minutes of palming to help the eyes, while the minimum amount of palming that helps with an exercise is fifteen seconds. We recommend thirty to forty-five seconds, but even fifteen seconds is useful for night walking as well as for other exercises. Breathe slowly, in deep breaths. Your pupils will have time to enlarge a bit. Then take your hands off and return to your other exercise.

From time to time, also stop to massage your eyebrows. Massage the right eyebrow from the bridge of your nose to your temple; then do the same thing on the left side. Massage your cheekbones and stretch the muscles of your cheekbones from nose to ear. Every time you firmly massage your cheekbone, you may find that more light penetrates your eyes and you experience a sensation of less squinting.

Step 7: Shifting

Shifting is an exercise designed to wake up your macula and helps develop the retina. In the retina, we have 126 million photoreceptors. Six million of them look at fine details, and 120 million of them look at the general picture. When we try to look at fine details, we can only see them well if we look at them centrally. We see them poorly, however, if we try to see them with our peripheral vision.

Shifting is all about moving your gaze from detail to detail. The eye has a natural tendency to shift from point to point. If you are the type of person who takes your time to see the beauty of the world and to look from detail to detail, you've already started this exercise.

I have recently brought out a simple device called "The Shifter." It has black and white stripes, and it's good for covering your strong eye from near. Wave your hand quickly to the side from time to time and, with your weaker eye, look at the black and white stripes. For those who see well, it's good to look at the small stripes; for those who see poorly, it's good to look at the big stripes because those stripes will help you to start shifting. Cover your eye with a small piece of paper. Wave your hand quickly to the side of your stronger eye. Look up and down at each line from beginning to end and from the end to the beginning. Close your eyes, visualize them, and look again. You don't look at them one by one; you simply look at each one of them up and down, up and down.

Figure 2.13. See the beauty of the world and look from detail to detail.

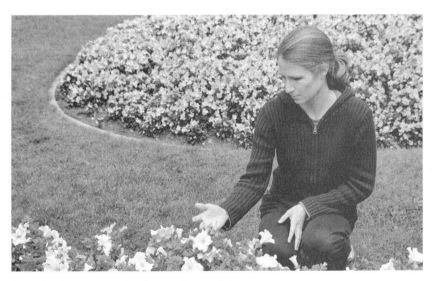

Figure 2.14. Let your eyes see whatever they see. Relax.

Later on you'll discover something precious: practically anything you look at that has patterns draws your eyes to look from point to point, up, down, and to the side. When you look that way, then your capacity to see those stripes becomes better, but then you can also count them better and move quicker. Then your eye will start to have very nice minute move-ments at all details it sees. But you want to be conscious of it and look from detail to detail: to see the frame of a window, and then the details of the window; to see the frame of a curtain, and then the details of the curtain; to see where a wall or closet begins and ends. Just like when you look at this particular shifter. It is not psychological but rather is a mental exercise in which you basically prepare your brain to look from detail to detail. That will wake up your macula.

Practicing Shifting

All you need to do is to open your eyes and to look at details, without contacts and without glasses. The beauty of this exercise, and the reason you can feel good about practicing it without glasses, is that you don't need to strain to try to see details clearly or perfectly. You just observe them. Let your eyes see whatever they see. Relax. If what you see is clear, that is wonderful. If what you see is fuzzy, that is wonderful, too. Enjoy the clarity, or relax and maybe start to enjoy the fuzziness.

After you observe the details of whatever you are looking at, close your eyes and visualize the margins and distances between details. Think about the contrast between those details. Have you ever thought about the pleasure of seeing contrast? Even if your general vision is fuzzy, when you notice the contrast between details, you start to activate the mechanism of perception that is so important when trying to establish a visual sense of your environment.

You can look at details from nearby, or you can look at details from afar. Go for a walk and look at a house. Then look down at the sidewalk. Look at a road, and then look at another house. From time to time, look into the distance for a short moment; then look back at the details of the street, the details of the road, and the details of the houses. Embrace the contrast.

Some people think the normal speed of the macula is as quick as seventy-two eye movements per second. The macula moves at great speed, and we want to help our eyes look from detail to detail rapidly, by doing it correctly and looking right. By shifting, looking at one detail and then looking at another, and examining the contrast between these details, we can reverse this habit and open up the tendency to truly look.

Look at More Details

Now that you are slowing down to notice the details of your environment, you can further vitalize your eyes by looking at even smaller and smaller details.

There was a time when I looked at details for thirteen hours a day, every day. I looked at windows and air conditioners. I looked at blinds and bricks. I would sometimes ask a friend of mine with better vision to look at the exact details that I was looking at and to describe them to me. My friend would always describe different details than the ones I saw, and this would make me want to study the details even more.

It is also helpful to get a group of people to stand and look at details together. As the group looks at an environment, say for example the waves on the ocean, they take turns describing what they see. Someone might describe a boat or a ship in the distance. Someone else might describe the boat's shape or color even more specifically. There could be a particular light on the horizon with different coloration. The larger the number of people describing these details, the more everyone can find new things to look for and discover new ways of seeing.

This happens instinctively with little kids because they get so excited when they respond to something they see. The same thing is true for us adults about details we look at: the more we look at details, the more stimulated we get. That sense of excitement in our eyes is apparent, and when anyone looks at our eyes, they see vitality in them. There is nothing as frozen as eyes that don't look, and there is nothing as alive as eyes that do look. When you look from point to point, you project that you have a sense of presence and attention.

The pleasure of looking at details is a form of unity with the world that nature gave us. The more we look on a regular basis, the less casual life is for us. Everything in life becomes interesting as we see all the differentiation within it.

I remember a biker who came to one of my classes in the 1980s. He rode his motorcycle from the peninsula, a forty-minute ride to our school. After studying for two and a half hours in a vision class, he went straight to Golden Gate Park just to watch the beautiful flowers in the arboretum, one by one. He looked at their petals and at their veins. He looked at their stems and at their leaves. He continued to find smaller and smaller details. The class had stimulated him to want to look at beauty.

I used to ask my daughter, Adar, to go to the beach with me. I would take along an eye chart, some tennis balls, and her glasses, which had an obstruction for her left eye—it was her stronger eye—to give her right eye a chance to work more. Since she almost always resisted going, I had to tempt her by suggesting that I would put her on my shoulders. Fortunately, she remembered that she had enjoyed being on my shoulders from the time she was a baby, so she would agree. When we arrived at the beach, she would do eye exercises as she looked at the waves and into the distance. Eventually, Adar began to notice that her reading of the chart had become much better and would always say, "Daddy, why did I resist coming to the beach? It's just so nice to be here."

On our way to the beach, we would stop from time to time, and I'd get her to look at signs. At times, we would stop at a flowerbed right near the beach, and I'd ask her to count two hundred petals with her weak right eye. As she counted, I would look at my watch and find the count had taken between fifty-five and fifty-nine seconds. This always surprised me because it seemed too quick. I also remember another time during her adolescence, while massaging and relaxing her in a dark room, I asked, "Adar, how many petals can you count in one minute?" She answered that she could count between thirty-five and forty. I said, "Adar,

I've timed you, and found that you can count two hundred of them in less than one minute." She replied, "But, Daddy, I can't follow my count." I answered, "That's exactly the point. You had counted automatically, and by exceeding normal speed with your counting, you engaged the macula in a function it already knows how to perform. You directed your macula to look."

So my daughter, whose lens was removed and whose cornea is small, was able to exceed all expectations about her vision by connecting her brain and her macula. Everyone can do the same, either with a healthy eye or with an eye that has some defect. Like my daughter, you too can make the connection between your brain and your maculae. You can move from detail to detail rapidly, and as a result, your vision can become as sharp as my daughter's vision had.

Find a lovely place to sit and look at beauty, to look from detail to detail of a beautiful thing. Once you gain this desire, the world will look beautiful to you and you will want to mobilize yourself. It is so important that you retain curiosity about details. As children, we have it naturally; as adults, we have to make an effort to give it our attention and our souls. It's wrong to be childish, because it is immature and it taxes you and the people around you, but it's wonderful to be childlike, to be unfrozen and in a state of perpetual awe.

If you were born with macular degeneration or have an inclination toward it, looking at details will slow it down and may even reverse it. Looking from detail to detail is the work of the macula. Your maculae become activated as many millions of cells start to come alive; their activity triggers activity in the brain. This activity, in turn, creates more synapses between the maculae and the brain, and the brain and the maculae. It's amazing how a small part of our body, the macula of the eye, can energize the whole body. It's also important that all of us strengthen our maculae so we will be able to see well for the hundred or more years that we could live

Shifting is one of the best habits to get into.

Figure 2.15. Find a lovely place to sit and look at beauty.

Read the Fine Print

People used to look at raindrops on leaves. They used to look at the fruit that matured on the tops of trees. Nowadays, people tend to just look at the big picture. We learn to try to look at whole pages of paragraphs, just to grab their contents without looking at the details.

In the past, we used to revere the written word. We used to read poetry. People used to look at every word and find something to respect. People used to read the same poem over and over again, and found new meaning each time they read it anew. Those times are over. These days, any poet who wants to try to live off poetry may just as well apply for welfare, because there's no way to make enough money by selling it. On the other hand, suspense stories and prose with low-level content sell, and because it's not extremely interesting when you look at it page by page, people don't mind skimming through a whole novel to get the gist of it. This only weakens the activity of the macula. It's the tragedy of the modern world that we don't really engage with great presence in whatever we're looking at.

The next exercise, therefore, is a good push in the opposite direction. Look at the page in this book with the different sizes of print, titled "Large and Small Print." Look at print size number 3, which is the size of normal print.

No one has perfect vision all the time, and our eyesight varies.

Bates checked hundreds of thousands of eyes

human and animal, young and old.

While his subjects slept, ate, got sick, underwent anesthesia,

posed for photos, did arithmetic, gazed at stars, played ball, and sewed on buttons,

Bates tagged after them and measured their vision.

The results surprised him.

Bad vision got worse, got a little better, had flashes of perfect vision.

Sleep often produced worse vision.

Normal eyes went nearsighted every time the subject told a lie.

Look at each letter slowly, in detail, as if you were writing it with your mind. Follow each part of each letter with your eyes, point by point, line by line. For example, if you see a Z, you can look at the lower line of the letter; then notice the middle line, and gradually take in the top line. Look even closer to see many different points in the bottom line, many points in the middle line, and many points in the upper line. Try to distinguish between parts of the Z, even though it is just one letter. Then continue to look at all the other different letters in this same way. Look at each different part of each letter as if you were writing them slowly with dark ink.

This way of looking utilizes the macula, the center of the retina, in the exact way you looked at the details in the world when you were an infant. At first, you may not have seen them well. But once you looked at whichever details you could see, you woke up the connection between the brain and the macula.

Now look at the largest print on the first of the two pages. Look from point to point on each letter in the large print. Then look back at the smaller print size and find whether you see them better than before. You can do this same exercise from two perspectives. You can start with small print and then look at larger print, or vice versa. In both ways, you should be able to reach the same results. You are training your brain to look at smaller areas than your normal tendency.

After you read the print in this way, look away from the page for a minute and see if you remember what you read. It is amazing how many people have absolutely no recollection of the text, or a very limited recollection.

I enjoy sharing this story about a student from a recent class I taught. He had lost nearly all vision in one of his eyes. The first day of the class, I put a patch over his stronger eye, or what he called his "seeing eye," and he had to be led around by another person. I had him read an eye chart standing two feet from it, and he could only read the eight largest letters. When I abruptly moved the chart away and ask him what he had just read, he did not remember even one letter out of the eight. I repeated this exercise three times, and he couldn't remember the letters he had just read. You have to understand that the eye is seeing, but the brain is interpreting what we see. The images we see are upside down and the brain turns them right side up. The brain pays little attention to our weaker eye, and we have to work to reconnect that communication between the weaker eye and the brain. I finally made some progress with my student after he remembered at least one letter. As a result he started to regain some vision in an eye that both he and his doctors had dismissed as being completely blind. The second day of wearing the patch, he still had to be led around, but he felt more confident. After successfully recalling what he had read on the chart, he walked undisturbed with an eye patch without being led around, and looked with the eye that he had dismissed as blind. He didn't see well yet, but he was not blind in that eye. If you have a weaker eye and a stronger eye, and the difference is not as great as my student's was, it is important for you to block the central vision of your stronger eye with just a small piece of paper taped to the bridge of your nose, wave your hand to the side rapidly to activate the periphery of the stronger eye, and read with the weaker eye, then close your eyes and try to remember what you read. Lack of memory in the weaker eye is too common. So, remembering what you read can make a big difference.

On a much smaller scale, what's amazing is when you start to remember part of what you read; even if you don't remember but just try to recollect it, you'll find that the vision in both eyes becomes much stronger.

This work with the macula can change you physically and spiritually. Quite often, we have a single-minded idea about the reality of life, when the reality of life actually has many levels and many variations. Looking at many details helps you experience the variations that both the physical and the psychological worlds have to offer.

The Ink Is Black, the Page Is White

For this exercise, with a small piece of paper taped to the bridge of your nose to block the central vision in your strong eye, look at an eye chart in bright sunlight, or under bright inside light. Look at the page and imagine that the black ink of the print is interrupting the white of the page. Slowly move your attention from letter to letter. Start with the largest print on the first line. Meanwhile, wave your hand quickly to the side of the stronger eye. This way, you're simultaneously working to increase the periphery of the stronger eye and improving the central vision of the weaker eye.

You are engaging your weaker eye in practice that it's not used to. Normally, the strong eye dominates. When there is stress on the visual system—and I would like to suggest that most of us, even those who have good vision, have some visual stress—the tendency of the system is to use the strong parts and suppress the weak ones. But this is unhealthy for us. It makes us work very hard to see. When you wave to the side of the strong eye and you look with the weaker eye, you wake up cells in the eye and in the brain that normally are not working. When you wake them up, there's a great relief, as there is more balance in the system, and no one group of cells works harder than the others.

Now close your eyes and imagine that the space is white and the ink is black, and remember a single letter you just saw. It will give you a sense that you are really looking at that letter. Say out loud, "The ink is black, the page is white." You don't need to wave your hand quickly while your eyes are closed, but you can imagine that you are waving your hand to the side of the strong eye while reading with the weaker eye. Then open your eyes and wave to the side of the strong eye and read the next line with the weaker eye. Now close your eyes and say out loud, three times, "The ink is black, the page is white." Then open your eyes and wave your hand quickly to the side and read the next line. Next, look away into the distance, and wave your hand quickly to the side of your head. Now look back at the fourth line without changing the distance at which you started; then close your eyes and visualize the letters again. Repeat the process for the last lines of text. Each time you close your eyes, say out loud, "The ink is black, the page is white." Or say the opposite: "The page is white and the ink is black."

When you finish doing all these movements, look back at the third line and see how clear it became. Then look back at the first line. You have trained your brain to look at smaller details with the eye that normally did not work as much as the other. In this way, you create equality in your brain, which takes away the stress from underusing the weaker eye and overusing the stronger eye.

You should see these results rather quickly. Most people are astounded at how much better they can see when they take the paper away from their eyes. For a timespan that could last for two seconds to several minutes, they can see the page in much greater clarity because they used their weaker eye.

Repeating this exercise two or three times a day for the first two months, and once a day for the next three months, will forge a whole new pathway in your brain, where the brain becomes accustomed to utilizing both eyes in unison.

Accompanied by other exercises that we will do, this will start to wake up the precious maculae in both eyes. This is relevant because the macula reflects what is in the universe. One of my workshop participants, a physician by profession, spoke like a poet, and his poetry resonated deeply within me and within the other workshop participants. He said, "The macula is like the sun, and the periphery is like all the stars around the sun. The farther you get from the sun, the less bright it is. The farther you get from the macula, the dimmer you see. But you can see with dim light."

He was absolutely right. The farther you get from the macula, the less you see bright light and clear details, but the more you see dim light and unlit details. There is a place for both the macula and the periphery. We need to use both. The macula can be stimulated by strong sunlight with the sunning exercise. It is stimulated by your thoughts and by your actions. The more you look at details, smaller details from nearby and smaller details from afar, the better you see.

Look far away right now. Look at a cloud. Look into the distance, just like you learned to do before. As you look far into the distance, you see clouds and mountains, buildings and sky. While you see clouds moving, or mountains on the horizon, wave your hand quickly to the side and look into the distance. Also, pay attention to smaller details than the ones you would normally see. Let's say you see the windows of a faraway building. Now close your eyes, and visualize the windows and their frames. Try to recall details within one single window. Then open your eyes and look from window to window. Do not strain to see. Take a look at the absolutely smallest details you could possibly see in one window, as long as you don't strain.

Now close your eyes and visualize a contrast. If you saw a white curtain with a black frame, visualize the differentiation of those colors. If you saw wrinkled curtains, close your eyes and visualize the difference between the wrinkles and the protruding parts; then look up and down that window. From there, start to look at all the rest of the windows. Moving from one to the other will activate your macula. Additionally, you don't lose the periphery and you pay attention to what you see with your weaker eye while waving your hand to the side of the stronger eye.

In most cases, a person's weaker eye for proximity is also his or her weaker eye for distance. Though with a minority of cases—but still a high percentage—it can be that one eye is stronger for seeing near, and the other eye is stronger for distance. If this is the case with you, do this exercise first with your eye that sees well from nearby; then do it with your eye that sees well from far off. This work can make a very big difference to you in that both eyes will participate more equally in whatever you're looking at. As you continue to look from afar, you will see that your eyes get sharper, just like from nearby. As you look at smaller details, the larger ones become clearer because your macula has gained function and can look with great speed from detail to detail. In fact, the speed is so great that you cannot notice.

You can also examine how well you see from mid-distance. Mid-distance is somewhere between four feet and fifteen feet. You can use the same "fist telescope" technique that was mentioned earlier to tell if one eye is stronger at mid-distance.

Comprehension Problems with the Weaker Eye

A third of those who have disparity between their eyes have comprehension problems with their weaker eye's reading, meaning that what they read with the weaker eye, they don't necessarily retain. This exercise works to correct the disparity.

I recommend blocking your strong eye with a small piece of paper taped to the bridge of your nose. Now wave your hand quickly to the side of the strong eye. Read three sentences with your weaker eye; then take the page away and, from memory, use a tape recorder or MP3 player, cell phone, or any other recording device to record yourself as you repeat what you read. Now play the recording back while reading along with the weaker eye. Eighty percent of those who do this realize that their retention of information is bad with the weaker eye.

If you have a partner to work with, keep reading the sentences to your partner as you recollect them, until you get the sentences right. This will help to build retention with your weaker eye. Before doing this exercise, be sure to palm for six minutes, in addition to sunning and working with both eyes; only then should you isolate the weaker eye.

Step 8: Blocking the Strong Eye

This next exercise, as physical as it is, can also give you a whole new mental outlook of the world. The best lighting in which to do this exercise is in sunlight or outdoors. Otherwise, very strong interior light will work if it makes it easy for you to see the letters.

Look at the page in front of you from a distance that is comfortable and easy to read. Wave your hand quickly to the side of your head, all the way above your forehead, to the side of your eyes and beneath them. You could also wave a colored piece of paper around, or a toy with different colors, or a stick with a ribbon, or anything else that draws your attention. Look centrally at the letters on the page while peripherally sensing the object that you wave. As a result you will be working both your periphery and center together. That will release your eye from strain. Your eyes, as I mentioned before, cannot strain if both eyes are being used together.

Whenever there is strain, it is because one eye is being used more than the other. This exercise can make a huge difference by helping you to integrate the center and the periphery. Anytime you are looking at something that you can't easily see, like a menu or a newspaper, wave your hands quickly to the side, and slowly but surely the letters will become clearer to you.

Now take the small piece of paper, approximately one inch by two inches, and tape it onto the bridge of your nose so it covers your stronger eye. To make sure you have done this correctly, close your weaker eye, and make sure you cannot see the chart with the stronger eye that is covered. Then wave to the side of your covered eye and read the page with your weaker eye.

Make no effort when you read with your weaker eye. Any effort that you make will slow down your progress in several ways. It will stop you from adopting the habit of looking with your weaker eye at small areas. If it is strenuous for you to look with your weaker eye, your instincts are going to try to prevent your progress. You only need to make one big effort: the effort to make no effort. This will become easier through relaxation.

You are now waving your hand to the side of your strong eye. Wave quickly. The wrist flips toward your ear, and you make sure that your hand does not move farther than your periphery can see. Your strong eye is truly looking straight at the paper, but the central vision of your strong eye is being put on hold for the moment. The periphery of the stronger eye is being fully used and, in fact, it may expand. You will be paying attention to a peripheral view that many people inhibit when they look centrally.

Be sure to relax your face. Your face relaxes when your jaw drops and you have a sense that the cheek is a bit longer. Relax your neck and create a sense that the neck is lengthening a bit. In fact, you can even imagine from time to time that a string lifts your head up and your neck is lengthening.

Keep waving your hand while reading with your weaker eye. Put the page at a distance where the print can be read with slight effort. Your job is to minimize the effort. The way to do this is to follow each letter as if you are spilling dark ink on it or painting it with a marker, as if you were writing it line by line, point by point. Observe the white of the page, around the letter and sometimes within the letter, and the black of the letter. When you remove the piece of paper, the two maculae will be working together without one suppressing the other.

Most farsightedness could be reduced and perhaps eliminated with this kind of exercise.

Cheap Sunglasses

Buy yourself some cheap sunglasses and remove the lens from the side that is your weak eye. Then cover the other lens with an opaque tape such as dark duct tape. Put the glasses on and, with your weaker eye, look into the distance.

Figure 2.16. The glasses block the central vision of your strong eye while encouraging the peripheral vision to expand.

After you have looked into the distance for a while, take a rubber ball or a tennis ball and play with that ball at a distance. (Have three balls available to do any and all exercises requiring a ball, so that you will have another on hand when one gets away from you.)

For example, you can look at a wall twenty feet away; then take the ball and throw it at the wall ten times and catch it. The ball may not return straight to your hands, but don't lose your patience; just keep playing with it. This exercise helps to develop the lens, and it also helps with central vision.

After doing this for a while, use the eye chart in this book. It is best to have two eye charts available: one ten-foot chart and one twenty-foot chart. The twenty-foot chart is especially good for those whose vision is poor. The ten-foot chart is for those whose eyes are stronger.

Stand five to ten feet away from the charts to look at the first two or three lines. Stand between ten and twenty feet away to see the top six lines, where you do not see the bottom four lines too well. Then take a

Figure 2.17. Take a ball and throw it so it hits the large letters (a). Tennis ball hits eye chart (b).

ball and throw it so it hits the large letters of the twenty-foot chart and one of the large letters of the ten-foot chart. Throw the ball and catch it. Do this fifteen times in a row. You may find that you can see an extra line on the eye chart, maybe even two additional lines. Take your glasses off and use both eyes. With both eyes, you most likely will see one to three lines better, and there will be a very nice feeling of clarity of vision through deep relaxation. You allowed the strong eye to rest and the lens of the weak eye to work fully. The lens became flat when the ball hit the chart, and round when the ball returned to your hand. And you let your macula work well from afar because the central vision works well when it looks at small details.

Next, you can work with the eye chart the same way in which you worked with the page in front of you. Put the piece of paper on the bridge of your nose to block the central vision of your strong eye. Wave to the side of your strong eye, while looking with your weaker eye at the print that you see clearly. For example, if it's easy for you to see the first letter

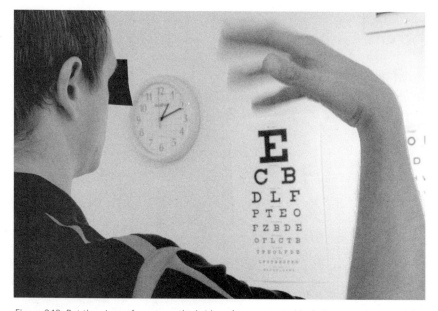

Figure 2.18. Put the piece of paper on the bridge of your nose to block the central vision of the strong eye.

or the first line, but it becomes progressively harder for you to see the second or the third line, then look at the first line, point by point and line by line. Do this as if you were spilling black ink on each one of the letters, and making them sharper by following the different parts of each letter.

Wave to the side, above, and below your strong eye. Make sure that the strong eye does not see any letter on the chart. (If you close your weaker eye, the paper should block the central vision of your strong eye, and your strong eye would not be able to see the chart.) When you wave your hand quickly to the side of your strong eye and you look with your weaker eye, you wake up the macula and strengthen it. This strengthens the nerve impulses and the muscles of the weaker eye, and it feels good.

Just as you did with the larger print, look at the smaller print while imagining that you are drawing the shapes of the letters. Many people then see the small print better. Look at the lowest line that you can see, which could be the third, fourth, or fifth line on the chart, as you wave your hand quickly to the side. Now look three lines below and look at the spaces between the letters. If you cannot see the spaces between the letters three lines below, look two lines below; if you cannot see the space between the letters two lines below, look one line below. Always look below your comfort zone at spaces between the print, even though you cannot read the print. Close your eyes and say to yourself, "The ink is black, the page is white," while imagining that your hand is waving on the other side. Saying this makes your brain engage with much smaller spaces from the distance that you can comfortably see the eye chart, whether it's five, ten, or twenty feet, depending on your vision.

You will then get engaged with that particular distance, and that engagement gets you to see well from that distance. Keep waving your hand on the side of your strong eye while looking at the print that you cannot really see. After looking from point to point in that print, look back at the line that you could see. Fifty percent of my workshop participants and private clients can see that line more clearly, and some of them could even see an extra line, or a few letters of the extra line, more clearly.

One particular optometrist, who took a workshop of mine, told me this was "eye-opening" for him (no pun intended). And indeed it was. When you take the paper off, you experience that with both eyes you can see a couple of lines below the ones that you saw before, for the two maculae are working together without one suppressing the other. The effort of looking is then diminished, the desire to look increases, and the other exercises that you started to do will work better for you. When you look from a distance, you will make no effort to look at details. They will come and go; slowly and gradually, you will see more and more of them, as far as the horizon and as close as forty yards away.

Look at Details One More Time

As I said earlier, the motivation to look at details is very important. It is nice to see adults wanting to look at something trivial, something that isn't necessary for life, like an animal walking, a beautiful garden, a sunset, or cloud formations. You can't pay your bills with gorgeous skies, but when you look at them in a meaningful way, you're engaging in something significant. When we were kids, we didn't judge anything because we were not capable of earning a living then. We looked at everything out of curiosity and, indeed, childhood vision is precious and great.

When we lose our curiosity, we lose much of our vision. Through inhibition and the demands of life, we learn to look at letters in order to gain content from them, and sometimes to see a page at a time, without looking at one single dot on that page. We observe other people only in order to understand what their expression means to us for a particular purpose or endeavor. By looking at a food shelf without paying attention to all that's on that shelf, just looking at the specific item that we need, we soon cut out 90 to 95 percent of the details that the world presents to us. The reason is that we know what we want far too well.

The problem is that we suppress the work of central vision and of the whole eye mechanism. The visual mechanism—the brain—does not pay attention to most details. The eye does the same thing. Many muscles get frozen: the ciliary muscles of the lens get frozen; the iris muscles of the pupils get frozen; and some of the external muscles get frozen as well, since they are not being used. Much of the retina is not working.

I will never forget the time I saw a father and his daughter looking at some print. She was fifteen and he was in his mid-forties. She could see print much smaller than he could. He could see down to the fifth-print level, and she could see down to the eighth. I said to him, "At your age, you could see exactly what she sees." After seeing hundreds of kids and how excellent their vision can be compared to the "normal" vision of adults, I could understand that childhood vision, even if it is less than normal, is much better than most adults' vision. The father said to me, "What have I been doing all my life? I've missed out on something very important." He had done important things in life: he was a surgeon, he had operated on people and saved lives, and he read books, but he did not pay attention to his own visual system; day by day, second by second, it decayed. It was clear to him and to me that if he could begin to be vigilant about his visual system and work with it, he could learn to improve his sight. Even after decreasing his visual acuity as much as he had, he was able to gain a lot of acuity that day, and saw better.

In the cases of people who have lost retinal cells, renewing an interest and appreciation of details can help them gain back much of their lost vision. Your curiosity and need to look at details increases with these exercises, and you will feel more alive. You will feel that you breathe better and meditate clearer as you go along in life.

Our work, therefore, is to wake ourselves up to look at details and to revive the dormant centers in our brain. Much of the potential we possess is latent and asleep. It's hidden from us because we adopt bad habits that we incorrectly think will work for us.

There is continuous debate these days about vision. One side believes that simply having normal visual function is sufficient. The other side believes that paying attention to your visual function and working on it constantly is just as important as its functioning. The second group is still a minority, but that minority is growing. If you are reading this book and practicing the exercises, you are in the minority that believes we should always work on improving our vision. If you are in the minority, you also believe in vitalizing our vision and giving it life.

Now you are armed with many eye exercises that can help you see better and feel better. Make time to do these exercises daily. The most important thing in life is to pay attention to the universe. The universe begins with you and your body. When you pay attention to your eyes, you'll be in better contact with the whole world. You'll also bring more circulation to your eyes and you'll feel better. Then you can help your own life, and find it will be easier for you to help the world.

Sometimes an exercise will work perfectly fine one day, and not the same way the next day. There are many reasons why this happens. For example, palming will work better if your shoulders are relaxed and worse if they have retained tension. Shifting will work much better if you are refreshed. Blinking will work much better if you have a good night's sleep and if you are relaxed at the time.

One sign that you're doing well is if you find yourself looking at details for no special reason: observing and not ever straining to see them, but always having a sense of all the details in the object you're looking at; you're enjoying the object or looking at it in total neutrality. If you find yourself breathing deeper and absorbing the world with greater joy, then all these exercises will carry themselves into your day-to-day life and become natural habits.

Step 9: Blink

In order to improve our awareness of blinking, and to receive all the benefits of blinking, we have to have individual control over each eyelid.

One great exercise is to simply open and close each lid separately. Another is to cover one eye with your palm; then concentrate on only opening and closing the other eye. Imagine that the eyelashes are doing all the work of opening and closing the eye.

If your eyelids feel dry or sore, you should either palm or just close your eyes for a while. A reliable way to rest your eyes is to put a warm towel over them and relax them. This will increase the blood flow to your eyes. If you have inflammation in your eyes, putting a cold towel on them will feel nice. Lying down with a warm towel over your eyes is great, especially if you can put a cold towel after that, because cold towels help the eyes in many ways. They help them become moister, and they help to de-inflame them because of extensive computer use. So one minute with a cold towel can really help the eyes quite a bit; however, warm and cold is the best combination, especially on a cool day. If you don't have time for warm and cold towels, just take a cold towel that was either two minutes in the freezer or fifteen minutes in the refrigerator.

Figure 2.19. Cover the right eyelid with your fingers right underneath the eyebrows, and blink with the other eye.

Through relaxation, you will discover a profound difference in your ability to blink. As you look at details, you will find yourself gently blinking. Your eyelids should feel weightless. For a fraction of a second, the eyelids close and then open; It will happen quickly. It will massage your eyeball and trigger moist and pleasant tearing. It will also trigger the widening and expanding of the pupils as you open and close your eyelids. Blinking should be very gentle and pleasant.

When you blink and your eyes feel refreshed, looking at details becomes easy. It sounds counterintuitive to many people, as the feeling is that blinking interferes with looking. Nevertheless, the rest you receive from closing your eyes for a brief moment helps you to move from detail to detail with greater ease. In fact, without that rest, the mind would have a hard time concentrating on any one point. The rest allows you to keep functioning with greater ease. Blinking massages your eyes and brings you more vitality. The desire and willingness to look gives your whole body more life. Relax your forehead. Relax your jaw. Relax your temple. Experience the wonderful sensation of vitality in all of your face, neck, chest, and upper body as you blink.

If you sleep well and feel refreshed, if you exercise gently, if you feel relaxed and sense that the blood flows better in your body, you will find yourself blinking with greater ease. And if you blink with greater ease, you will find yourself relaxed and that the blood flows better throughout your whole body. Blinking influences, reflexively, the sense of relaxation and movement in the body. If the jaw drops and doesn't crunch, then the shoulders drop and do not elevate, and the pelvis becomes loose—just from blinking gently, softly, and continuously at a rate of twenty-two to twenty-five blinks per minute. Blinking and looking at fine details is something that most children do automatically. It gives you a sense of youthful energy.

A good blinking exercise is to move your head in a rotating motion in each direction for a total of five minutes, very gently. Perform this motion in medium-size circles while blinking in order to bring more blood to the head, which, in turn, will make blinking easier.

Another wonderful exercise is to put one hand underneath the other, while gently pressing with your head against your hands, and moving your head in a rotating motion in both directions. When you put one hand underneath the other, your hands are steady and there's the sense that you are bringing much more blood to your face.

A great way to prepare for blinking is to blink in a dark room, where it's easier for the eyes to open and close. Blink three or four hundred times in the dark. Then massage your eyelids very gently. With a very light touch, stretch the eyelid from the eyebrows to the eyelashes several times;

then, you will start to be ready for one of the most difficult exercises in this book.

To do this exercise, first gently cover the right eyelid with your fingers right underneath the eyebrows, and blink with the other eye. When you blink, remember to think how the eyelashes are doing the work of blinking. Since your hand is covering your right eye, you can feel how much your eyelid moves when you blink your other eye. The goal here is to be able to blink the uncovered eye without experiencing any movement at all in the covered eye. This is very difficult and requires much practice. You must touch gently the covered eyelid as well as the forehead while you try to blink only one eye. Massage your forehead and temples gently with your fingertips. Cover your closed right eyelid with your fingertips. Touch the right eyelid very gently. Imagine that the eyelashes of the left eye are moving the eyelid and that the forehead is not working, because it is in the muscles in the middle of the forehead where the two eyes merge and unite when one suppresses the other. On a tissue level, you want one not to suppress the other. Now repeat the exercise while covering your left eye.

If you contract your face in order to blink, you teach your brain that the muscle that blinks is too weak to do it for itself, and it needs to borrow the forehead muscle. But if you loosen up the forehead and temples and skin rolls of your scalp, from the occipital area to the frontal area, you will find that it's easier for your eyelids to be independent. It's so important for us to remind ourselves that light eyelids are eyelids that have healthy circulation. It's amazing how much your sense of well-being improves when your eyelids are light. There is less fatigue all over the body. It is astonishing how tight your face, neck, chest, and upper body are if your eyelids are heavy.

Stroke your eyelids about six or seven times. Then cover one eyelid with your fingers in such a way that the fingertips are under the eyebrows. Do not put your hand on your forehead, because then you will not feel the eyelid. Just underneath the cushions of your fingers you will feel the eyelid, and you will feel how much it moves when you blink.

Blinking will help you develop your peripheral vision, and help you remember not to strain your eyes.

Step 10: Vision and Body

The health of the eyes is intertwined completely with the overall health of the entire body. Blood flow in particular has everything to do with muscular health, cardiovascular health, and relaxation. The following exercises will help you to maintain the health of your entire body while you continue to work on improving your eyes.

Walking Correctly

Walking is a wonderful exercise to stay fit and active. It is a low impact way of exercising and gets your blood flowing. But it is important to pay attention to how you are walking.

Make sure that you are walking heel to toe, with correct posture: spine straight, chin up, and shoulders back. Do not slouch. Do not let your head droop. Look where you are walking so that your neck is not stiff. Now relax. Do not tense your shoulders; just make sure they are not drooping forward or down. Remember not to strain. Being tense while walking is never good. Relax and enjoy the fresh air and exercise.

It is also good sometimes to walk backward and even sideways.

Rest Your Eyes

We must rest our eyes completely. For 1,500 years, Tibetan yogis have made it a point to spend extended periods of time sitting in dark caves and meditating on the color black. When they exited the caves, their vision was incredibly good. Just think how much they stretched their pupils.

In the Jewish culture, we meditate on the color blue since we believe, for some reason, that black is the color of sadness, a funeral color. But it isn't sad. In fact, it's a wonderful color, one of total rest for your optic nerve.

Today, because of city lights, we strain by not having fully stretched pupils. When you stretch your muscles, you can then contract them much better also. For example, if you stretch your hamstrings, you will feel much lighter when you walk. The same thing happens to your pupils; it's just that the response is not as quick, so we don't feel it.

The pupil has two round muscles. One muscle widens the pupil, and its collaborator contracts the pupil. To properly stretch both muscles, you need to sun and to night walk because, unless your pupil can expand all the way, it will never be able to contract all the way. The more you can constrict your pupil, the clearer your vision will be. Whether your vision is only 20/400 (about 10 percent of normal vision) or 20/40 (85 percent of normal vision), you will end up improving your capacity to see better with constricted pupils.

Quite often, after having a long nighttime walk in an area that doesn't have much light, people who see 20/40 will improve their vision to 20/20. After this, city lights may suddenly start to be a bother. We are learning that city lights disturb the pupils by not allowing them to expand all the way. Of course, city lights aren't completely bad because they can help us find our way. We go to coffee shops as a result of having city lights. We can travel with ease as a result of having city lights. But we never experience the pupillary expansion that is so necessary for better vision. The muscle that expands the pupils simply does not work all the way.

After fifty minutes of night walking in the park, the muscle expands all the way, and the whole face and neck relax. The next day, it's much easier to contract these muscles. You will respond much better to the sunning exercise if there is also expansion from looking in the dark.

One way to help your pupils is to do many exercises in a very dark room. To make a room completely dark, close your curtains at night; then play in there with a glow-in-the-dark ball. Relax as you do it. When your eyes open wide in the dark, you will experience relaxation all over your body. Then try this with the piece of paper mentioned before, taped from your forehead down to your chin. Throwing the ball from hand to hand above your head can also help your eyes to stretch. You will find that your eyes rotate much easier in the dark. When throwing the ball from hand to hand above your head, the ball goes above the head and, for one moment, the ball disappears. When people ask me why this exercise is good, I tell them to put the ball in front of their right eye and close it. They don't see the ball. I ask them to put the ball in front of their left eye and close it, and again they don't see the ball. So, in fact, when the ball gets to the left hand, the right eye does not see it. When the ball gets to the right hand, the left eye does not see it. Therefore, the eyes start gaining independence, which leads to much better vision for both of them.

If your eyelids are fatigued or your eyes hurt, and it is a hot day, lie down and put a cold towel over your eyes for about three or four minutes periodically throughout the day. If it's a cold day, then put a hot towel over your eyes. I always found this a great vacation from life. I also found that whenever I worked with patients in San Francisco, where we often have cold air and fog near the ocean, they relaxed themselves and improved their progress if we put hot towels over their faces for a while. Sometimes, lying down and closing your eyes for four or five minutes can make a very big difference.

Deep relaxation of the eyes, and proper contraction of the pupils in the dark, will lead to more relaxation in normal life and can help us to maintain good vision for life.

The Power of Breath

When you practice blinking, one of the automatic reflexes is slow, deep breathing. The slower your breathing is, the more relaxed you are.

The best way to breathe is slowly in and out through the nose. When you breathe, you want to feel your abdomen expanding when you inhale and shrinking when you exhale. You want to feel your ribs and chest expanding when you breathe in, and shrinking when you breathe out. Proper breathing encourages a sense of calmness and relaxation in which blinking and looking at details becomes easy and natural from moment to moment.

When you breathe, you feel warmth in your hands and feet. You also feel balanced throughout your whole body. When you breathe deeply, light becomes easy for you to absorb.

So let your abdomen and your ribs expand, but also feel your back expanding with each inhalation, and shrinking with each exhalation. When we look with ease from detail to detail while blinking with ease, breathing slowly and deeply, and when we become adjusted to strong light, our vision comes alive.

Loosen Your Neck

You can loosen your neck in many different ways. One is simply to look into the distance while you stand erect. Do not let your head move forward. When you're standing erect, there is a ligament that holds your neck straight, just like there is a ligament that holds your lens flat when you look far into a distance. This is a wonderful position for the body.

Since the normal tendency for most people is to bend forward, usually the neck becomes tight. From time to time, stand erect and look far into

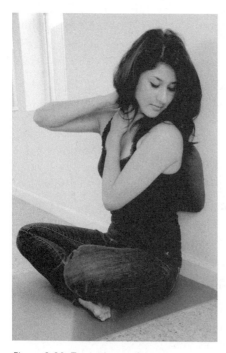

the distance, and you will maintain a soft neck that will not need any treatment; this will also bring more and more blood flow into your head. Using this technique, you will prevent many problems that relate to poor blood flow to the head.

Now, sit in your room on the floor with your back against the wall, with a small pillow that creates an arch in the middle of your back. Put your head against the wall and rotate your head from side to side. As you do this, stretch your neck. Breathe deeply and slowly. Tap with your fingertips on your neck, all the way from the base of your skull to your shoulder, back and forth.

Figure 2.20. Tap with your fingertips on your neck, all the way from the base of your skull to your shoulder, back and forth.

Now, for a brief moment, put your hand on the side of your chin and stretch your neck even farther to the left side; then stretch farther to the right side, while tapping up and down your neck to loosen the muscles. Do not continuously push your head. You will then find that the neck is stretching and, when you move your head from side to side, that it moves slightly better.

You do not need to do this exercise for more than ten minutes per day. Even so, it will be very valuable in preparing your body for other exercises in this book, because more blood to your head means less pressure in your eyes. And the pressure in your eyes, if abnormal, can cause problems. More blood to your head also means that you have refreshed eyes, and refreshed eyes tend to respond much better to these eye exercises.

More blood to the head has all these benefits I've mentioned and a great many more. It has absolutely no side effects, will make you feel refreshed, and will help you to be alert. It will help you to do what you want, while seeing at ease and seeing well. You will find that moving your eyes from side to side becomes much easier for you when more blood flows to your head, and all that can happen only with a loose neck.

Activity always leads to relaxation. When I was blind, I strained to see. Looking took away the strain, but I see many legally blind people who strain to see all the time. In fact, as they start to look at details, shifting without straining to see, they see them better. So, the more you look, the less you strain. Even though it's counterintuitive to many people, shifting is a very relaxing process. If you achieve shifting through all your waking hours, you'll find that your eyes become more and more relaxed. They look from detail to detail and they relax. Consequently, the whole body will relax.

Another relaxation exercise is to lie on your back with knees bent and hands to your sides. Now roll from side to side. Your hand will push you to roll to the opposite side. After you roll to the right, push with your left hand, and you roll to the right. After you roll to the left, push with your right hand, and you roll to the left. It is good to push with the back of the hand. Do this about one hundred times every day, before meals, for several months, and it will help your neck while increasing the blood flow to your head.

Another wonderful exercise is to sit up, interlace your fingers, stretch out your arms in front of you, and rotate them in a complete circle, in their entire range of motion, whatever that is for you. Visualize that your fingertips are leading the motion. The full movement of the arms loosens up your shoulders. Also, rotate your wrists. The looser your wrists are, the looser your shoulders become.

Figure 2.21. Interlace your fingers, stretch your arms out in front of you, and rotate them in a complete circle in both directions.

Figure 2.22. Now point your palms outward while moving your shoulders in a rotating motion in both directions. Circle your arms up.

For the past 150 years, we've had the tendency not to lift our arms all the way. Nowadays, many men and women wear jackets that restrict the movements of their arms. That stiff look of immobile shoulders has been around for too long.

Our ancestors used to climb trees and lifted their arms upward on a regular basis. We don't, and we're paying a very dear price for it, because not lifting our arms restricts blood flow to the hands, head, and eyes. These days, our fingers are very stiff. We write, we type, we drive, and we constantly contract our fingers. Musicians, sign language interpreters, and massage therapists like me tend to contract their fingers even more. We don't balance this movement with enough extension. Many workplace injuries and arthritic conditions happen because of stiffness in the wrist and fingers.

Interlace your fingers and point your palms outward while moving your arms in a rotating motion in both directions. This position helps you to stretch your hands and prevents lots of other problems. If you feel a nice stretch in your forearm, you have done your job. I remember a woman who took my class and had such poor circulation in her hands that they looked green. When she practiced stretching her hands and wrists, and moving her shoulders in a rotating motion, however, they became pink.

Stretch Your Eye Muscles

Here's a wonderful way to stretch your external eye muscles and relax your neck: put a long piece of nose-width paper, from your forehead to your chin, and throw a ball from hand to hand above your head, back and forth.

A student of mine named Melissa was in a terrible accident, where a Suburban pickup truck ran over her body and head, breaking many of her skull bones. Consequently, she was subjected to more than twenty surgeries on her face. One of the surgeries was on her deep orbit, and the recovery from it was very difficult. She developed extreme double vision and neck pain. When we put the small, medium, and large pieces of paper between her eyes, she saw well peripherally, but she saw double below and above those papers; her neck kept hurting as well. When we placed the big piece of paper from her forehead to her chin, and she threw the balls from hand to hand above her head, her neck stopped hurting, at first temporarily, then for the long term.

This practice of putting a long piece of paper from forehead to chin has become known as the Melissa Exercise. You simply tape a piece of paper to your forehead; then tape the bottom of the paper to your chin, and do exercises while wearing this paper. It may not immediately feel as much of a neck relief to you as it did to Melissa, because your eyes may not see double and you may not experience that extreme difference. Nevertheless, it may feel like a great relief for you from the strain of one eye that controls the other; this relief immediately leads to better vision for more than 60 percent of the people who do this exercise.

With the Melissa paper on your face, throw a ball from hand to hand above your head for five to ten minutes. You will see the ball in your right hand with your right eye, and when the ball crosses in front of your face, you will see it with your left eye as you catch it with your left hand. Only one eye can see the ball at one time. If you have access to a trampoline, it is wonderful to do this exercise on it while you bounce. Throw the ball from hand to hand above your head, allowing each eye to work separately as you try to catch the ball.

Figure 2.23. The Melissa Exercise.

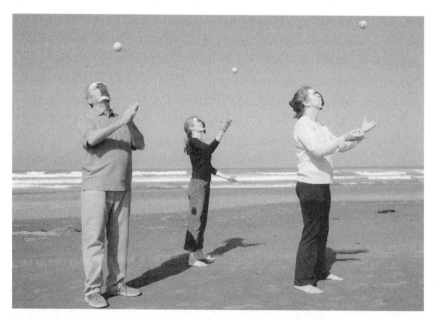

Figure 2.24. Throw a ball from hand to hand above your head while the paper is taped from your forehead to your chin.

There are many other variations of the Melissa Exercise that we will cover elsewhere in this book, but this is the basic starting point: throwing a ball from hand to hand above your head while wearing the Melissa paper taped to your forehead and your chin.

You may find that this eye-hand coordination, with a clear divider between your two eyes, can make a big difference and can help you relax your eyes. Keep doing the shifting exercise, which will also stimulate the macula. When you are refreshed, the macula works better, and all other parts of the eye work better as well.

Enjoy the View

Often, pleasant scenery appears in front of us—faraway places with beautiful views. But even people who go on vacation are entrenched in the habit of not looking. They will only spend a few minutes, here and there, actually looking at the view. Then they will go on to deal with their vacation plans and work-related issues involving computers. A reason for this is that they are not used to looking at the beauty that attracts our vision on a daily basis.

Some people do not have anything beautiful to look at in their workplace. Nor do they have anything beautiful to look at in their residence. But most people in the world do have access to beautiful places to look at somewhere in their lives: a nice garden, beautiful plants, lovely pictures, and even changing clouds.

Develop the daily habit of looking at something pleasant. We should devote twenty minutes a day, divided into four-minute increments, during which we spend looking at something beautiful. It could be combined with the looking into the distance exercise, or it could be apart from it. Spend a few minutes every single day looking at beautiful scenery, and it will slowly instill in you the desire to look at details. So, when you go for a vacation, instead of spending twenty minutes looking at nice details in nature, you may end up spending two or three hours doing just that, and still enjoying yourself.

We are creatures of habit. Whatever we do now will perpetuate what we will do later. Create new habits of looking at details: first with your lenses, then without your lenses, then with reduced lenses, then again with-

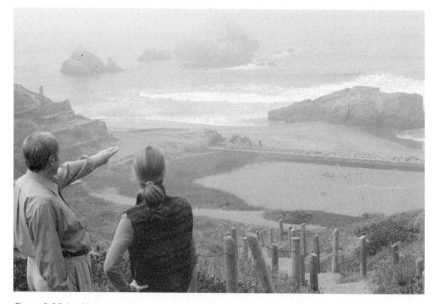

Figure 2.25. Looking at the distance relaxes the eyes if you don't strain to see.

out your lenses, then maybe with pinhole glasses that help the pupillary contraction, and finally without lenses or glasses at all. If we enjoy looking at details, we will develop a skill that is lost by modern life, and that skill is the ultimate fortress of strength for our visual systems.

If you have vibrant, healthy, and mobile eyes, as you look at objects, you will also relax your whole body, which will feel vibrant and thus looser and more mobile. Because the eyes lead the body, the body's posture arranges itself around the way the eyes see. Therefore, making your eyes more alive can trigger your whole body to come alive.

If you focus on your breathing and visualize expansion and contraction, you mimic the movement of the whole universe, which is in constant movement, expanding and shrinking. When you begin to sense this and move in that direction, it can give you a pleasurable relaxing sensation that you may never have had before. If you combine the visualization of blackness with the expansion and contraction of your body, you start to have a sense of an inner rhythm that you never had before.

Repetition of these exercises gives you a pleasant sense of relaxation that augments your sleep, but the benefits go much deeper. When your conscious brain learns to relax, not only will it relax when you palm, it will relax *anytime* you look. And that is exactly what you want to do: consciously relax, so your subconscious will start to work in a whole new way.

Don't Squint

Your tendency to squint is one of the highest hurdles on the path to vision improvement. Squinting is a manifestation of physical and mental resistance toward improvement and change. If you do not squint your eyes much in the light, your brain demands the pupils to contract; when they do, your vision becomes much clearer. If you do not squint when you read, you will start to look with a soft eye at the print on the page.

Ready to Move On

I would like to congratulate you if you have earnestly worked on yourself using all the principles and the exercises we've discussed so far, because it means you are devoted to your health and to your life. And who is going to help you if not yourself?

There is an old Jewish proverb: "if not now, when?" If I am not going to take care of myself, then who will? It is an illusion to think that others can do better than you can for yourself. So continue to practice with my suggestions, and you will feel the difference. Your vision will improve, and you will maintain your vision for life.

Chapter 3

Computer Use and Relieving Built-Up Fatigue

When working at a computer terminal, it's critical to be aware of your position, the lighting, and your overall surroundings. First of all, you should sit at a distance from which you can comfortably read the screen. There should be adequate lighting (natural light is best), but it should not be shining directly into your eyes; nor should it be reflecting off the screen, creating glare. Finally, the computer itself should be positioned where you can easily gaze into the distance: next to a window or a long hallway are good locations.

You can use the features of a computer to your benefit by following data as it appears on the screen or by visually keeping track of the movement of your fingers across the keyboard. Look at the actual shapes of the letters you are typing and be aware of the spaces between them.

Often, however, when we work at computers, we create an "invisible strain" that we don't really feel. This is the worst kind because if you don't recognize the strain, you will do nothing about it. And if you are actually straining, then by the end of a day of computer use, your eyes may be red and you will be unnecessarily fatigued.

So, what is it that actually makes you strain as you look at a computer screen? First is the weariness of looking from so close. If you look into the distance three times a day for eight minutes, it can help to alleviate this. Not everyone, however, has that amount of time, so even twice a day would suffice. This can occur before you start to work, during the time you're working, or at the end of the work day, if your eyes are not too tired. Our suggestion is that you divide it into four: ten minutes before you start to work, six minutes after one hour of working, four minutes after two and a half hours, and six minutes after five hours of working. Twenty to twenty-five minutes of distance viewing during six hours or more in from of a computer is mandatory to keep your eyes healthy and stress-free, providing you also do the other exercises. The main thing is not to strain: do not try to *see* the distance; instead, *scan* the distance. From time to time, use the obstructive lenses described in step 8 in chapter 2 to obstruct the eye that sees better from far away, even if the other eye sees better from near. Then take the glasses off and keep looking into the distance.

Every half hour that you use a computer, you should do something different and pay attention to your eyes, even if it's for a very short moment. If you focus on the rush of information coming from your monitor for very long, it's easy to disregard your peripheral vision. When this happens, your central vision becomes overtaxed, a situation that may contribute to glaucoma or lead to loss of clear vision. It's imperative to provide your central cells with some rest by stimulating your peripheral cells. You can accomplish this by doing the peripheral vision exercises, which will enable you to notice the periphery more: you acknowledge the floor, the wall, the ceiling, and your general work environment. When the periphery is being used, you won't tense your eyes as much.

We suggest taping a small piece of paper between your eyes, waving your hands to the side, and rocking forward and backward for a short moment. If you don't have a small piece of paper, close your right eye

Figure 3.1. It is imperative to provide your central cells with some rest by stimulating your peripheral cells.

and wave your hands quickly in opposite directions: one is up and one down, one is at right and one at left, while you are looking forward. Then close the left eye and do the same. This practice doesn't have to last for more than a minute, so it won't interfere with your work, but it will stop your stress in front of a computer.

The long swing can also work wonders because it gets you away from your computer terminal and forces you to do something physical with your entire body along with your eyes. Even if you have only a few minutes to do this, there will be a noticeable improvement in your vision when you return to your computer. The long swing is when you stand looking at your finger and move your body from side to side, thinking everything is moving in the opposite direction of your finger. Blink softly. You don't need to do it for more than a minute to relax your eyes and keep working. Read more about the long swing in step 1 in chapter 2.

It is also helpful to do the Melissa Exercise every day for five minutes. Place it anywhere in your day when your eyes are not so tired that they won't respond to an exercise. In this way, fatigue does not accumulate. You can do it during your workday or outside your workday, but do it every day. The Melissa Exercise is when you put a long strip of paper from your forehead to your chin over your nose and take a ball and throw it from hand to hand, as described in more detail in the section on cross-sightedness in chapter 5. It causes independence of the eyes and takes away strain.

Palming for a minimum of six minutes could also be beneficial at some point in your workday, preferably after not more than an hour of sitting at your computer. Palming, described in detail in step 6 in chapter 2, is when you rub your hands, put them over the eyes orbits very gently, with your elbows on the computer desk, preferably with a pillow, and focus on your breathing while relaxing your eyes. If you make palming an intrinsic part of your daily routine, it will help your eyes to recover from any strain they are undergoing. As your day progresses, you should alternate among all of these exercises in order to obtain the most beneficial results.

Throughout your entire workday, be sure to pay attention to the periphery as well as the fact that your two eyes are looking. From time to time, as you are reading the computer screen, put a small piece of paper in front of your nose, covering the strong eye. Then wave your hand to the side of the strong eye and read with your weaker eye. Close your eyes and try to remember the last line you read, and say it to yourself twice. This helps because sometimes the brain will remember only what you read with the stronger eye, and this will force you to read with both eyes.

While working, it's a good practice to look away from the computer for fifteen seconds every half hour and to work on your peripheral vision for one minute. Put a program on your computer to remind you every half an hour to work on your eyes. When your day is entirely over, it's good

to finish up with a ritual of three minutes of peripheral vision exercises
and one minute of doing the long swing. By doing this, the drawbacks
of computer work will not affect you as much; in fact, you may even be
encouraged to exercise your eyes more.

There are basically two problems that result from using a computer.
One is that we are just not meant to stare at a computer for eight hours
a day. Our ancestors did not do it, and through them we have developed
the kind of eyes that we currently possess. Nowadays, however, nearsightedness is increasing at an astounding rate. What worried William
Bates about schoolchildren in New York in the 1920s was that 6 percent
of them were nearsighted. Today, 48 percent of kids who attend school in
the United States are nearsighted. Sadly, the numbers are even higher in
other places: in Hong Kong, it is 62 percent; in Taiwan, 84 percent. The
entire world needs to understand the implications. While computers alone
may not account for these results, looking from near for long stretches of
time is partially responsible. This mode of working tempts us not to use
our periphery, which triggers nearsightedness in the first place.

The other difficulty is that pixels have unique properties, and it's
harder for the eye to see them, even though we don't sense it at the time.
The cumulative effect over a period of hours of computer use is substantial. Hence it is important to take our eyes away from the screen periodically and do these exercises. It is also essential to blink frequently yet
gently as we are working. Not only will this break the fixation of staring
at your computer screen, which contributes to eyestrain, it also serves
to moisten the eyes and to reduce tension in the muscles around them.
Burning, inflamed, or itchy eyes will eventually be alleviated by blinking.

From time to time, especially when you feel you are not responding to
any of the exercises, massage around the eye orbits from the bridge of the
nose to the temples and from the nose to the ears. Relax yourself, even if
it means only ten strokes (about twenty seconds) of this, which can really
remove the accumulated fatigue. If you're working on a hot day, you can
get invisible inflammation in your eyes. Lie down once a day with a cold,
damp towel around your eyes.

You need to have zero tolerance for building up unnoticed fatigue.
First, you need to be aware of its existence; then you need to remove the

fatigue as you progress through your day. The detrimental thing about reading from a computer screen is that we have incorrectly learned to read only the document in front of us, and not to pay attention to our eyes. If we have bloodshot eyes, we go to an ophthalmologist and get eye drops, thinking that fatigue does not adversely affect the eyes. But once it begins to accumulate, nothing will go right with your vision. It can be prevented by managing the fatigue.

It's important to take a day off sometimes. On that day, don't use a computer; instead, do some eye exercises. It's also beneficial to take time off during each day not to look at a computer screen; designate times for using your computer and times when you won't be using it. Naturally, this will vary with the individual, and whereas some people prefer to enjoy their day, using their computers only at night, others will prefer just the opposite. Once you have decided on the hours you will not be working, you can revive yourself from computer use by doing other things and by paying more attention to everything it kept you from using, like your peripheral vision and your weaker eye. Otherwise, by looking from near, you can strain one eye; looking from far, you can strain the other.

Value your eyes as much as you value the material with which you are working. Similarly, value your breath just as much as you value your project. The moment you make these decisions, the computer will never harm your eyes. If your decision is to ignore them, however, the computer can seriously harm your eyes. Don't believe people who tell you that a computer can't damage your eyes—that advice alone is damaging.

Chapter 4

Improving and Correcting
Errors of Refraction

In this chapter you will find specific exercise programs I recommend for the treatment and, at times, the reversal of vision problems related to errors of refraction. These include myopia, hyperopia, presbyopia, and astigmatism. Although this chapter specifically focuses on errors of refraction, the exercises discussed here will aid in the treatment of many conditions discussed in chapters 5 and 6. These include cross-sightedness, cataracts, diabetes, glaucoma, optic neuritis, detached retinas, vitreous detachment, macular degeneration, and retinitis pigmentosa.

If you are currently under the care of a physician who is open to a holistic approach to healing, I encourage you to share this information with him or her. Together you will be able to monitor your progress and adapt my suggestions to your particular condition. These exercises are intended to work in conjunction with whatever else you are doing to heal and to maintain your vision.

As I mentioned in the preface of this book, many doctors are quick to prescribe chemicals and even surgery to correct all problems, including vision problems, and will often discourage you from believing that your condition can ever return to normal, regardless of whatever efforts you might be willing to make.

What, after all, is the definition of healing? Healing does not always mean an instantaneous cure, a total reversal of every ailment. Sometimes that happens but, more often, true healing comes in small steps. True healing is simply an improvement, however minor, within the parameters of what is possible given the circumstances of your life. It is important to make comparisons only with yourself. If you can improve, however slightly, from where you are today, give yourself the validation of acknowledging that small success. Build upon it and celebrate it. Cele-

brate every small accomplishment along the way, and remember where
you started.

I cannot stress enough how much faith I have in people's ability to heal
themselves through the diligent practice of these programs. My personal
experience of working with myself, my children, and with thousands of
patients and students has taught me that improvement is possible, and
that the benefits of these exercises are tangible and well within your reach.

Suggestions for Using This Part of the Book

First, make sure you have familiarized yourself with the basic exercises
explained in chapter 2. I will refer back to them again and again. Now
turn to the section in this chapter that addresses your particular vision
condition. Follow the exercises I recommend for at least the time periods I suggest in each section. Most importantly, make a commitment
to incorporate these exercises into every aspect of your daily routine. I
may recommend six minutes of palming or ten minutes of sunning, but
this is only a starting point, the bare minimum. Ideally, instead of setting
aside one part of your day to do these exercises, you will find moments
throughout your day to exercise so that the improvement of your vision is
always at the forefront of your mind. Don't stop being conscious of your
eyes and the ways in which they function throughout the day. Never stop
looking at details.

Think of this part of the book as a starting point. As with muscular
exercise, the best program is not simply to work out for thirty minutes
a day, three times a week, while being sedentary the rest of the time. The
best idea is to incorporate movement and physical exercise into every
aspect of your life. Walk throughout the day. Take the stairs instead of
the elevator. Do subtle movements and easy stretches throughout the
day. This way, you are always exercising and always aware of your
physical condition.

The same principle is important here. Start with my recommended
time periods for these exercises, but learn to always find time throughout
your day to palm, to sun, and to look at details. Accordingly, awareness
of your vision will become ubiquitous, and will be a priority to you no

matter what else you are engaged in throughout the days and weeks of your normal life.

Make a long-term commitment to the program and take time out to measure your progress regularly. Do not give up. Do not set unrealistic expectations of instantaneous healing. Take every success, no matter how small, and build upon it. Keep a journal of your progress and your feelings along the way.

If, at any point, you feel as though the exercises are taking you in the wrong direction or are not creating the benefits you desire, it is possible you could benefit from additional therapy. There are classes all the time at my School for Self-Healing in San Francisco, and I also offer off-campus lectures and therapy sessions around the world. I encourage you to research possible opportunities to work with me or with one of my trained practitioners, if you believe it could benefit you in your quest for better vision.

Where Do Corrective Lenses Fit into These Exercises?

Ideally, as long as it doesn't cause you stress or strain, you will practice improving your vision without wearing your lenses, at least part of the time. Once you are a month into doing your exercises, go to a friendly optometrist who doesn't oppose your working on your eyes and ask for a pair of glasses that corrects them to 20/40, which is 80 percent of 20/20. When your eyes see better with those new lenses, go back and get a new prescription at 20/40. Getting used to the lower prescriptions will build your eyesight.

Now, some people with very severe myopia (nearsightedness), of 20/500 or lesser vision, should have three different pairs of lenses: the 20/20 glasses to drive with on foggy nights for safety; the 20/40 glasses to walk around with in the daytime; and 20/80 glasses with which to challenge themselves while walking around in a familiar environment. In most cases, after two months of this, you will be able to see 20/20 through the 20/40 glasses. Then you can go back to the optometrist and change back to 20/40 again, the new 20/40. We expect you to reduce 2 diopters a year and to see better all the time.

At a certain point, when you feel comfortable walking outdoors without glasses, we suggest you get a pair of pinhole glasses and put them in your pocket. Look at people's faces and signs up close without glasses. When you are at a distance where the signs or faces are not as clear,

however, put on the pinhole glasses and use them to read signs or to recognize faces.

Also, you can use the pinhole glasses while reading. Before you put on the pinhole glasses, as you read, look into the distance, scan the horizon and look from point to point. Next, look at points in the distance that are a little bit closer to you, and then look at points that are even closer than the ones

Figure 4.1. Pinhole glasses.

you've just looked at. Do this for no less than four minutes. After that, reading through the pinholes will be easy, at least for the next fifteen or twenty minutes. First, look far into the distance for a few minutes to rest your eyes; just look without trying to see anything in particular. Then read without glasses for fifteen or twenty minutes and look into the distance again. Next, read with pinholes for a half hour and look into the distance again. Finally, read with your regular prescription. This is not a perfect exercise for everyone, but it can be adjusted to fit your situation. What should never be compromised is that you should never strain your eyes to read.

Pay attention to your individual abilities; if you can hold on longer with the pinholes, that's fine. What you want is simple: to gradually transition out of the continuous use of your glasses.

If your myopia (nearsightedness) is not severe, that is, if you see 20/200 or better, my suggestion is to walk everywhere without glasses, unless you drive or have a specific safety reason that requires you to wear glasses. Meanwhile, keep the pinhole glasses in your pocket. When you see a sign that you can read, but with difficulty, or that you can hardly read but can follow some of the shapes, put on the pinhole glasses and look at the sign again. Often, when one puts on the pinhole glasses, they can see the sign better. Pinhole glasses work with two-thirds of people, but not with everyone. Pinhole glasses also work with most of my students, but they do not work with me. They either work for you or they don't. Since they are not expensive, however, it is worth your while to try them and find out.

Correcting Nearsightedness and Farsightedness

Imagine that you are using a projector to show a film. If you have placed the screen too far away from the projector, farther than the focal point of the lens, the image will be blurry. To someone with myopia (nearsightedness), this is how the world looks. Things nearby are clear, but things faraway are fuzzy. With hyperopia, it is as if the screen has been placed too close to the projector. Things close by are fuzzy, but things farther away are clear. With presbyopia, the lens is too stiff, so things close to you are out of focus because the lens is not round enough for the picture to fall clearly on the retina.

Myopia (Nearsightedness)

Myopia is a vision disorder in which a person can clearly see nearby objects while objects in the distance appear blurry. Also called nearsightedness, myopia occurs when the eyeball has become too elongated, and light entering the eye isn't focused correctly; this is what causes distant objects to appear blurry.

High myopia is an extreme case of nearsightedness requiring more than 8 diopters of correction, and progresses consistently. Though you see well with correction, the eyeball continues to become longer and longer, which causes the retina to become thin, thus risking detachment. This detachment deprives the photoreceptors of vital nutrients and can lead to blindness. There are many other severe problems besides retinal detachment, such as glaucoma and macular degeneration, which can occur if your vision does not improve without glasses. As your vision improves, the eyeball regains its normal round shape.

This is why my work is so critical. You can see it as physical therapy for the eye. And in this case, it's very important. If you decrease the length of the eyeball, even by half a millimeter, and prevent the continuation of the high myopia, then you may be able to prevent the expected retinal detachment and, prior to it, vitreous detachment. This is where the vitreous detaches from the retina, causing bleeding and floaters. If you already had some detachments, it may help prevent more. So while physicians are so eager to fix the detachment when it happens (they may be right in doing so), and they simply tell you that vitreous detachment is not damaging in most cases (and they're right about that as well), sometimes they remove the vitreous if they feel that a detachment could strategically damage important parts of your retina. This is like a case of lattice retinal degeneration, where they remove the vitreous in order to avoid a detachment that will take away the macula and cause a macular hole.

So we work on reducing your myopia, and that myopia can essentially be reduced with eye exercises. For that reason, doing the eye exercises is critical for anyone who has 8 diopters or more. We expect you to improve 2 diopters per year for the first two years, and 1.5 diopters in the next year, and then 1 diopter farther on. Slowly but surely you will improve your vision until you will not need your glasses. We hope you will greatly improve from the experience, but even if you improve by 0.5 diopters, the result could be amazing for the rest of your life.

Even people who wear three pairs of glasses (a 20/80, a 20/40, and a 20/20) due to poor vision have to find moments to be without their glasses, and will then see better through all of them. Perhaps this will be when the light is very clear, like in your backyard, or on a familiar street, or in your home if there is good light. The 20/80 and the 20/40 will both be clearer, and the 20/20 will be sharp. The less you wear your glasses, if you don't put great strain into seeing, the better you will see through your glasses—and, in time, decrease their prescription. Eventually, you will be able to see well without them.

We can see how one problem leads to another if we don't take care all the time to improve our eyes.

Beneficial exercises for correcting myopia include shifting, palming, peripheral exercises, reading with pinhole glasses, and night walking. Devote at least one hour a day to these exercises, and remember not to pack the entire hour into just one part of the day. Find time throughout the day to work on your vision. Try a session of night walking once a week. If you live in an environment where it is not safe to night walk, you may wish to substitute walking around and moving in a dark room for forty-five minutes; this can wake up the rods through movement, although there is really no perfect substitute for walking outdoors at night.

Once you begin to experience improvement, you may want to increase the recommended time periods for each exercise. This is a good idea and can lead to even more improvement in your vision. In truth, my recommended hour of exercise should be considered a minimum starting point. If you have very severe myopia, you may want to start with an hour a day and, as you experience improvement, you can move up to two hours a day or more. An hour one day might seem extensive if you are busy, but on another day it may not be a big deal to spend several hours.

Exercise Program for Myopia

Night Walking: 45 minutes, once a week.

Shifting: 10 minutes daily for the first two months; 5 minutes daily after that, and throughout the day, with 30 seconds here and 30 seconds there. You should find minutes here and there to pay attention to details until it becomes subconscious. From time to time, you can check on yourself and see that you are constantly looking from detail to detail, all the time progressing to smaller ones.

Palming: 20 minutes daily.

Peripheral Exercises: 10 minutes daily.

Bouncing the Ball: an extra exercise for myopia.

For this last exercise you will need a tennis ball, an eye chart, and your sunglasses, with its lenses popped out and the strong eye's lens obstructed with duct tape. You should have your eye chart posted on the wall at eye level. Basically, what you are going to do is put the glasses on and throw the tennis ball at a line on the eye chart, and try to catch the ball again. But it is actually a little more complicated than that.

Stand in front of the eye chart at a distance from which you can read the top three lines well, the middle lines with more difficulty, and the bottom lines as being completely fuzzy. This is the correct distance from

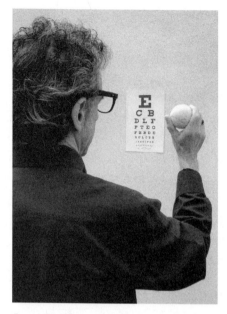

Figure 4.2. Wear your obstruction glasses covering the strong eye and throw the ball at the chart.

which you have the opportunity to make improvement. You should not be closer than three feet away, but whatever distance beyond three feet is comfortable for you should be okay. It is important not to judge yourself harshly about what distance is comfortable for you. If five feet is your distance, work to achieve improvement at five feet; if seven feet is your comfortable distance, work to achieve improvement at seven feet. Remember that you are seeking something very personal and should only compare yourself to yourself.

So, put on your cheap sunglasses, the ones with the lenses taken out, and the strong eye's side blocked with a dark tape. Pick up the tennis ball and extend your hand out toward the eye chart. Aim the ball at one of the largest letters on the chart. Retract and extend your arm several times, as though you were taking careful aim. Visualize that the ball is hitting the chart and flying back into your hand. Now throw the ball at the chart and try to catch it again.

Repeat this exercise from all the different angles you can. Throw the ball at an angle from one side; throw it at an angle from the other side. Throw it overhand and underhand. Throw it with a lob; then throw it straight out in front of you. Now take the glasses off and look at the chart again.

I assume that when you put on the obstructive lens, if you see the first three lines with both eyes, you may only see the big letter or the first two lines with the weaker eye. Some of you will still see the first three lines, except fuzzier with the weaker eye.

After throwing the ball in all the directions we described, when you take the glasses off—if you're one of the 80 percent of the people in my workshop, or I can compare you to one of that 80 percent—most likely you will see the fourth line, and a letter or two of the fifth line. Then you can look at the sixth line, which you could not read, and look at the spaces between the letters. You could even try looking at the seventh, and if you don't make any effort, look at the eighth. And look at the spaces between the letters, then close your eyes and remember the letters and the spaces. Often in my workshop, the whole group says "letter, space," several times. So if you have eight letters in a line, you say "letter" eight times and "space" seven times, to make it really clear to you that you are seeing the letters and the spaces in your mind. If it is a line in which you can still see the spaces between the letters, but the letters themselves are indistinguishable from one another, you could say "character, space." Then look back at the fourth line, and it may appear much clearer; look then at the fifth line, and you may be able to read most of it. At that point, you know that you had a temporary improvement that could repeat itself more than half the times that you return to look at the chart. If the fifth line became clearer, but not every letter there is clear, close your eyes and say, "The ink is black, the page is white." Say it five times, open your eyes and look at the print again. The whole idea is not to strain by trying to identify details of each separate letter, but instead only to identify the relationship between them, that one is a space and one is a letter.

Now put on the glasses again and throw the ball back at the eye chart. Repeating this exercise often yields positive temporary results, and gradually over time, for many people, it improves the ability to see lower lines on the chart.

A variation can be done while running in place. For this variation, attach a medium strip of black paper to the bridge of your nose so it obstructs your strong eye. Now run in place and bounce the ball on the eye chart, catching it again if you can. With your other hand, wave your hand quickly in the periphery of your strong eye. You wave your hand quickly to the side of the stronger eye so it can only pay attention to the periphery, providing that you are looking straight at the paper that obstructs it. Your job is to never lose track of the hand that is being waved to the side. The important thing here is to get your two eyes working together. The reason that you run in place is to keep yourself moving, so you will not freeze your gaze. Breaking the tendency to freeze is the beginning of better vision.

The next step is to run in place with the paper obstructing your strong eye, and to throw the ball back and forth with another person. Do not put the paper in the middle of your eyes. Make sure you are obstructing the strong eye, so that you are working on both the periphery of the strong eye and the central vision of the weaker eye.

When you look at the eye chart before beginning this exercise, look at the lowest visible line, where you can see most of the letters but not all of them. Pick a letter you can see clearly. Close your eyes, visualize the letter, and say it out loud. For example, if it is a Z that you can see clearly, say, "The Z looks clear. The Z looks wonderful. The Z is black and the page is white." This is just to appreciate what you see. Enjoy the fact that you see the letter clearly. Instead of saying, "I don't see clearly," you are saying, "This is what I do see, and it is wonderful." This is positive reinforcement, but you are doing it in a very tangible way. The Z *is* wonderful! Even if it looks fuzzy, you enjoy the way it looks anyway. Respect what you have and work with it.

I have met quite a few people who compare their vision without glasses to their vision with glasses, and they are not enjoying the vision they have. Allowing yourself to enjoy the vision you have, however, is where the healing begins. It's like the old adage that the one who is rich is the one who is happy with his fair share. You're talking about a field in which people are so emotional and so aware of what isn't there, without ever really being grateful with what they can actually produce. Say, "The O is great! The A is great!"

Now look back at the chart and see if you can identify more letters. If you can, be grateful because the very fact that you can breaks the concept that many doctors are stuck in—that the eyes cannot improve—which is bogus. The improvement may be temporary, but it will show you the possibility that daily repetition of this exercise will help your myopia to improve over time.

While practicing this exercise, you must experience definite improvement from the distance that you have designated for yourself before you change your distance. Some people are tempted to change their distance too quickly. For example, they see really well from five feet, after not seeing well from five feet, so they move quickly to ten feet. Nevertheless, you have to understand that the eye of a nearsighted person is very rigid, and the mind of a nearsighted person is fixated with the vision they have.

So, if you improve from five feet, enjoy your improvement. Get used to the clarity from that distance. Experience it and love it. Enjoy the fact that you see better and that you can measure your improvement. Stay at that distance for six months before you increase the distance by two feet. When you experience improvement from your new distance, stay there for six months; then increase three more feet. The gradual improvement is the permanent one. It needs daily work, and you can't neglect it.

An additional exercise is to look at the eye chart from a distance that is comfortable for you. Look at a line that you can almost read; then move up two lines from there to letters that you can easily read, but that are not sharp. Now take a sheet of paper and make an entire page of letters that size. Create for yourself two pages of random letters, with anywhere from twelve to twenty letters on the page. If your vision is highly challenged, use as many sheets of paper together to give yourself at least twelve different letters to look at. Now hang your paper next to the chart, read it from the exact same distance you read the chart before, and allow your eyes to become comfortable focusing at that distance. To ensure you are truly focusing on that letter size, read them from left to right and right to left, up, down, and diagonally, so that you don't simply recite the letters. This exercise is best done with direct sunlight on the page. You can also do this same exercise wearing the obstruction glasses and looking with only the weaker eye. Reestablish the letter size that is comfortable, but not sharp, with the weaker eye. Repeat the steps above, then return to your original page with both eyes.

Look at the letters that you printed, then look again at the shifter. With great patience, look up and down every stripe, both black and white. If you are very, very nearsighted, look at the thicker stripes; if you are not so nearsighted, look at the thinner stripes, and then look back at the chart and see if your weaker eye is tracing the letters well. Sometimes, with both eyes you can see the chart from the distance you stood, but with the weaker eye you can no longer see even two lines above, and that's okay.

You look at the shifter and you look at bigger letters, and then you look at the letters that you printed and you see the space between them. You see the white within them, and maybe you can even guess some of them, and then you look again with both eyes. And 80 percent of people see the letters much more clearly for a while.

You have to keep working until the results are satisfactory. Sometimes you may take a break from exercises, or sometimes you will change them. Instead of always doing one program, you can deviate to keep your mind fresh and to keep engaged in your exercises; this way you will not get bored. Then you will go back to the original exercises. Be patient with yourself, because all vision improvement has to do with inner patience.

Looking at a distance is also a very important exercise for myopia. Walk at least once a day, with an obstructive lens over your strong eye, and look at medium distance to far distance. Wave your hand quickly to the side of the covered strong eye, and sometimes tap very, very gently with your fingers on the covered lens, just to acknowledge and notice it. You can play ball, or simply look at windows and trees or clouds. From a near distance, put the small piece of paper on the bridge of your nose, in front of your strong eye, and wave your hand quickly to the side of the strong eye. You can read, or look at nearby objects, also indoors, only using the small obstruction paper. The reason is, you need maximum periphery with your stronger eye for the weaker eye to not strain. So when you can spend hours on your vision, look at a distance with both eyes open, then put the obstructive lens on your strong eye for fifteen seconds, and then take it off. Wave your hands quickly to the side and close your eyes, and visualize that you are seeing the distance with both eyes. Then visualize you are seeing it only with the weaker eye. Then visualize you are seeing it only with the stronger eye, and again visualize that you are seeing it with both eyes. Open your eyes, and wave your hands quickly to the side so as to not lose the periphery. Get your hands closer to your face and farther from your face. All the way apart and slowly closer together, and again all the way apart while you look at the periphery. Do not tire your arms. After a while, simply massage around the eye orbits or do nothing. But keep looking at a distance for as many as four minutes at a time or six minutes at a time, up to twenty minutes at a time. Do not tire your eyes looking at a distance, and this will relax your eyes greatly.

I found that people who bounce—for example on a trampoline or run in place—can see better after they do so because of the additional blood flow to the head. So repeat all these exercises after bouncing for a short while, like two minutes at a time. Kids respond to it better than adults, but adults respond to it as well. The bouncing or the running in place should be a challenge but not too big of a challenge. If you are way overweight, don't bounce so much; instead, run in place. If you are light and thin, bounce on a big trampoline and then do the chart work if you have one in front of you; if not, you can bounce on the floor and run quickly, and you'll find right there and then that the eye exercises are more effective.

An Additional Note about Myopia

Most people with myopia have a good focal point somewhere. Let's say someone sees well from a foot away. That person should do the eye exercises involving eye charts and pictures, and anything that can help with looking at details and shifting, from a distance of thirteen inches, then from fourteen inches. One inch at a time will make it possible to develop vision from afar. So, inch away from the reading chart or the page with large and small print; an inch away is just like looking at an eye chart from two feet away, and every inch you get ahead enables you to read a smaller line of type. And remember to do it in strong light, like sunlight, or indoors with a light of two hundred watts or more. You will find that the light improves your capacity to see smaller details from a slightly farther distance. That's all you want to achieve: to see slightly better and better all the time. The gradual improvement is the permanent one, but it needs daily work. You can't neglect it; you have to keep working. You might change the exercises or focus on different areas, but you must keep working. Be aware that there are eye charts in the back of the book with which you can thoroughly practice. Keep one for measurement, which you will not memorize, and practice with the rest.

Hyperopia (Farsightedness)

Hyperopia is a condition in which you have a short eyeball. With hyperopia, because the eyeball is short, a picture coming into the eye falls behind the retina. So when it hits the retina, it does not appear clearly. Since the eyeball is short, you may see fuzzy from nearby or from far away, and you may not have a good focal point from either distance.

The normal prescription for myopia is minus lenses (reduction). Hyperopia, as well as presbyopia, before being cured by natural vision improvement exercises, is corrected with plus lenses (magnification). Also, plus lenses are prescribed when your eye's lenses—which are inner magnifiers—were removed as a result of being born with cataracts. All can be helped with natural vision improvement exercises.

Many children before the age of six have hyperopia, where they see well from afar but not so well from nearby. Children who are born with cataracts and had their lenses removed will have their vision corrected with plus glasses or plus contact lenses, which act like a magnifying lens. So, it is the same for children as for adults: because our lens is a magnifying lens, their lens will also be a magnifying lens. And it is very important to remember that when you teach your child to read before the age of six, you may cause eyestrain. Before this age, it is better for children to look at pictures and shapes than it is to look at letters. If you do teach your child how to read early, use large print.

Conventional wisdom says that it is normal for one to be farsighted when he or she hits their mid-forties. In fact, people don't even call it an eye problem. Instead, they say it's a part of the aging process. This is an amazing misconception, and one that I personally cannot accept. Is arthritis or types 2 and 3 diabetes part of the aging process? Truthfully, if you develop the correct habits, you can live to the end of your life without developing any of these disorders.

And there is also a way to prevent farsightedness. Be very flexible with your neck, be flexible with your head, and practice the following exercise program every day. Remember: don't simply set aside one part of the day to work on your eyes. Find time throughout your day to work on your eyes so these exercises can become a part of your lifestyle, a constant memory through which you are always consciously working on your vision.

Exercise Program for Hyperopia: 90–120 Minutes a Day

Sunning: 20 minutes daily.

Peripheral Exercises: Pay attention to the periphery all the time, and do at least 20 minutes of intensive peripheral exercises each day.

Palming: 18 minutes, preferably half an hour daily, in 6- to 10-minute intervals, unless you are very relaxed, and then it is in 10- to 20-minute intervals.

Look Far into the Distance: 20 minutes daily.

Extreme Close-Up: 20 minutes daily.

The Melissa Exercise: 10 minutes daily.

Extreme Close-Up: An Extra Exercise for Hyperopia

Prior to doing this exercise, make sure you look far into the distance; then palm for at least six minutes. Because you have hyperopia, looking at nearby objects is undesirable for you, and you have become accustomed to looking at objects from afar. So now you should train yourself to do the exact opposite.

Find an object that is pleasant to look at, like a flower or a painting. Stand a foot away from your chosen object. Now wave your hands quickly to the side of your face, putting your face very close to the object (about two or three inches away), and look at different details. Then go back to standing a foot away, and determine if you can see the object any better. If you find that you can, it means you have temporarily relaxed the lens muscles, and that your lens has temporarily become more flexible and less rigid. In terms of presbyopia, it also means that you may have elongated the eyeball temporarily.

Now, cover one eye and rotate your eyes in all directions: follow your thumb, look at your thumbnail until it disappears; then bring it back to where you see it; again, let it disappear on the side. So if you look with the left eye, look at your left thumbnail, and at a certain point, when your right eye would have seen it, it will disappear. Bring your thumb back to

Figure 4.3. Cover one eye and rotate the eye that is open in all directions. Follow your thumb in all directions.

where you can see it and move it back and forth as you stretch the eye, and you will find that you can stretch the eye more and more. Do exactly the same thing with the right eye, and then move both eyes in a rotating motion again.

Next, move both eyes in a rotating motion.

Look up, look to one side, look down, and look to the other side.

Figure 4.4. Move your eyes in a rotating motion.

Now put your thumb and your index finger on the bridge of your nose. Slide them up and down the length of your nose while looking at your nails. Look at the two nails from two sides as you look up and down. When you look at your nails, you slide them slowly all the way from the bridge of your nose to the tip of your nose, and then all the way from the tip of your nose to the bridge of your nose. As you look at your nails, you will find that you are straining quite a bit. Most (meaning 99.9 percent) people cannot see the two nails at once when they move them up and down their nose.

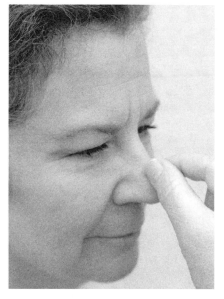

Figure 4.5. Place your thumb and index finger on the bridge of your nose and watch your nails as you slide your fingers up and down your nose.

Use both fingers and shift your eyes quickly from one nail to the other and hopefully within a month or two you will be able to see both nails at once. So, you start with your two fingers above the bridge of your nose at an area where the bridge of your nose meets your forehead. You then move them one centimeter below your nose, and you keep going up and down, up and down, trying to watch the nails. After two minutes of this, look back at the nearby object from one foot away, and see whether it appears clearer to you now. Now look far into the distance for two minutes; then look back at the object in front of you again. Your eyes should have relaxed significantly.

Now that you have discovered which of your eyes is dominant seeing from near in "Discovering Your Strong Eye" in step 2 in chapter 2, tape a small piece of paper to the bridge of your nose, covering only the central vision of the stronger eye, wave your hand to the side of that eye, and then put the other hand very close to the other eye, as if you can see the lines of your palm. Do it in the strongest daylight or sunlight for ten slow breaths, and then take the paper away from the bridge of your nose. Your vision will be way better.

Next, take the page with large and small print, make a copy of it, and put the very, very large print right in front of your eyelashes. Move from one letter to the next by moving the paper to see the letters one at a time, and then move backward from one letter to the next, and then look at them upside down while your eyelashes are touching the page. It's going to be a very strenuous effort for you. Don't forget to wave it to the side of your covered, strong eye, so you keep seeing the periphery with that eye as you read the letters using the central vision of your weaker eye. Then take the paper off, blink, and look back at the paper normally. You will see much better.

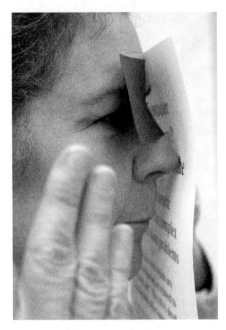

Figure 4.6. Move from one letter to the next and wave your hand to the side of your strong eye.

Be aware that you are exercising. This is not a normal way to use your eyes. These exercises are also great for presbyopia.

Correcting Presbyopia

Warning: We have to understand that with presbyopia and hyperopia, there could also be astigmatism. So before or while you do these exercises, it is good to do the astigmatism exercises. Especially good is the exercise where you wave the page with large print in front of your eyes while looking at the eye chart. This really takes away the astigmatism.

Hyperopia and presbyopia are similar conditions. The difference is that presbyopia is a stiffening of the lens that occurs through use of the eyes, usually when someone is around forty years old. This condition makes it difficult to focus on nearby objects. Often, people who develop presbyopia start to wear reading glasses to help them focus on books and newspapers or other objects at close range. Hyperopia, on the other hand, is a short eyeball, a condition you are either born with or that occurs because of a modification of the eyes. In my opinion, it's because of poor or incorrect use.

The prevailing concept among most doctors is that once your lens is stiff, it can never become flexible again. This is the only reason why people don't work for more flexibility: they have been incorrectly told that it is impossible.

If you are able to arrest that concept and understand that your lens is all-powerful and capable of responding to these exercises, you will never be presbyopic again. Furthermore, you will maintain good reading vision into your mid-nineties or early hundreds.

For presbyopia we do vigorous exercises to look from near, and we have to rest the eyes by looking from far away. Normally it's easy for the presbyopic person to see things from far away. So, for example, I suggest for people with presbyopia to look at the ocean, at boats, at the waves coming to shore. You can also look at buildings or at the sky, and only then do the exercise we suggest for presbyopia. You look where the letters are not very clear but clear enough to read. Do the exercises we mention and do them diligently. By first looking at a distance and then looking at the letters from amazingly near, you will find that those letters are easier to read. You have to repeat it several times so the lens of your eye will become more flexible and then reading will be easier, especially in strong light.

Exercise Program for Presbyopia:
90–120 Minutes a Day

Work mostly outdoors at first. As you improve, work in gradually dimmer and dimmer light. And remember: don't squint!

Extreme Close-Up (from the hyperopia section): 10 minutes daily.
Peripheral Exercises (using the obstructive lenses): 10 minutes daily.
Bouncing the Ball (from the myopia section): 5 minutes daily.
Look Far into the Distance: 20 minutes daily, divided into two or three sessions.
Rotate the Eyes: 5 minutes daily.

Extreme Close-up (from the previous section on hyperopia): at least 20 minutes daily.

Massage around the Eyes: 10 minutes daily.

Extra Exercises for Presbyopia: 10 minutes daily.

The Melissa Exercise: 10 minutes daily.

It is important to reiterate the necessity to work on these exercises throughout your day. Even though I suggest 10 minutes of a particular exercise, it is better to do a few minutes here and a few minutes there to get into the habit of constantly working on improving your eyesight.

Extra Exercise 1 for Presbyopia: Blinking One Eye

In this exercise, you are going to practice blinking with each eye separately.

As I have mentioned before, when you close one eye at a time, your brain learns to allow the two eyes to function independently. The way to do this is to close one eye as if you were blinking with it; then cover it with your hand. Now take your hand off your eye and open it. Repeat this 100 times for each eye. Afterward, you will find that you have a bit more control with each eye. Although you do this as a concentrated exercise, remember to blink gently throughout the whole day.

Extra Exercise 2 for Presbyopia: Reading in Dim Light

First, practice reading in dimmer and dimmer light each time you read. Now have someone turn the lights on and off while you are trying to read. Next, practice some of your other exercises, like reading big and small print or bouncing a ball in dim light as well.

This practice will improve your vision in strong light within four months. It will also improve your vision in normal light within ten months, and will help you to see in dim light within sixteen months. No longer will you be dependent on glasses, which will be a great thing for you.

Extra Exercise 3 for Presbyopia: Look Near, Look Far

For this exercise, you will want to find something that it is very pleasant for you to look at, like a beautiful picture. Look very closely at the object. Now put a small piece of black paper on the bridge of your nose so it obstructs your strong eye. Then look closely at the picture while waving your hand in the periphery of your strong eye. Next, look away from the picture and far into the distance. Continue to wave your hand quickly in the periphery of your strong eye. Now look back at the picture again, this time close-up. Take the paper off your nose and look back into the distance with both eyes. Now look back at the picture close in front of you with both eyes. You may be able to notice more details this time. It would then be a good idea to palm for six minutes in order to relax your eyes. Remember to stop and relax anytime you are feeling strained. The object is not to strain but to relax your eyes, your neck, and your body.

Extra Exercise 4 for Presbyopia: Creating Controlled Stress on the Ciliary Muscle for Strength

1

What is computer vision syndrome? It is, according to the

2

American Optometric Association, "the complex of eye and vision problems

3

related to near work which are experienced during or related to computer use." The AOA developed this diagnosis after seeing

4

an increase in the number of patients requiring eye exams due to symptoms they experienced at the computer. The visual stress of working at computers can bring on nearsightedness (myopia) or make it worse, and can also worsen middle-aged farsightedness (presbyopia).

5

CVS is a repetitive strain injury. One muscle that is strained is the ciliary muscle, a muscle within the eye that changes the shape of the lens to determine the focus. Pixels, which make up the images we see on the computer screen, are bright in the middle and blurry on the edges;

6

the brain is unable to determine a focal length for pixels, and endlessly attempts to do so. The iris, a muscle within the eye that regulates the amount of light that enters the eye, is strained by inappropriate lighting and glare, which are often a problem with computer work, and the result is light sensitivity.

1

LARGE AND SMALL PRINT

Nothing is more surprising than change, when it arrives—but nothing is more predictable. When we get into our forties, most of us begin to have trouble reading small print. The newspaper becomes easier to read if we hold it out at arm's length.

2

LARGE AND SMALL PRINT

People who have always had 20/20 vision start to walk around with reading glasses in shirt pockets or hanging from a cord around their necks, and those who are nearsighted switch to bifocals. Doctors assure us that it's a common change at middle age; our ciliary muscles, which change the shape of the lens to focus the eye for near vision, weaken, and the lenses become stiffer as we age. What they don't tell us is that the lenses can get even worse—eventually we can get cataracts, the biggest cause of blindness throughout the world.

3

LARGE AND SMALL PRINT

It's not a lack of compassion that causes eye doctors to go on prescribing ever-thicker glasses without warning us of the dangers that lie ahead. They simply feel that it's hopeless, that our eyes can only get worse. Schneider and other vision improvement teachers believe that eyes can also get better. They say that ophthalmologists are seeing only one end of a continuous spectrum—whether you see nothing more than lights and shadows or have vision that is more acute than 20/20, you're somewhere on the continuum, and change in either direction is possible.

4

LARGE AND SMALL PRINT

Even when your eyes are working hardest, trying to make out small print in dim light, for example, they need to function out of a sense of relaxation; this is the bottom line. This is why upper body massage is so important for good eye care.

The eye's own built-in massage, blinking, gets curtailed with the frozen stare that is the hallmark of bad vision.

Blinking bathes and refreshes the eye, gives it intermittent rest, and promotes flexible use—for example, if you're blinking while walking, your eyes open each time to slightly different scenes.

Unbalanced vision/movement patterns create tension in the eyes and poor vision; thus, massage therapists can help clients improve their eyesight by working with them on posture. Midback, shoulder, and head posture are especially important—if the head is habitually tilted forward, for example, the brain assumes that distance vision is limited, and it does indeed get worse.

5

LARGE AND SMALL PRINT

The eye exercises teach relaxed use:

To adjust the eye through relaxation to all intensities of light;

To balance the use of both eyes together. Uneven use creates enormous tension; the domination of the stronger eye needs to be limited, and the weaker eye needs to be strengthened. If one eye, or part of one eye, is damaged—even to the point where it can do no more than register the presence of light—it should be stimulated; the stronger eye will relax, and its vision will improve when the brain senses greater balance;

To balance central with peripheral vision. By habitually gazing at books or computer screens for hours at a stretch, we tend to ignore peripheral visual information until the periphery actually shrinks;

To create a flexible, fluid eye so that the eyes move easily between near and far;

To stop freezing the gaze and shift the eye easily from one small detail to another, lightly skimming the world like a butterfly.

6

LARGE AND SMALL PRINT

You may feel that wearing glasses relaxes your eyes; some people say they feel undressed and unready to meet the world without them. They do create problems—they teach us that without their help, we can only see poorly. They also tend to make us lose peripheral vision, since we are used to limiting our reality to what is visible within their frames.

7

LARGE AND SMALL PRINT

Of all the eye exercises, palming—a visualization of blackness coupled with awareness of soft, expansive deep breathing—is the most important. A meditation in its own right, it can relax the eyes, quiet the senses, and bring calm to an overwrought nervous system. Palming can be done passively to clients, or you can massage their necks and shoulders while they palm. It is a powerful tool. Long palming sessions can be harmful with glaucoma. Massage is a good substitute. Combined with breathing and movement exercises, massage can create a deep awareness of upper-body tension, especially around the eyes, so that the client learns to release it.

8

LARGE AND SMALL PRINT

The "cone" cells of the retina supply daytime color vision in sharply realized detail. To supply central vision, the normally sighted eye is continuously moving, easily and accurately, from one small, clear detail to another—the behavior called shifting. The periphery is supplied by "rod" cells. Although our vision is incredibly high-resolution—we have 100 to 200 million rods and cones—we don't all see all the parts of the visual field equally well. With normal vision, we see our small detail best, in a field of increasing haziness. Accepting this can be hard for near-sighted people, who often find blurriness unpleasant. Because the brain fills in what we expect to see, the entire periphery appears to have color, but it doesn't. Try standing in an unfamiliar room with many small colored objects, looking straight ahead; you wont be able to identify the colors at the edges of your visual field.

Ideally, this exercise should be done outdoors on a bright day, with sunlight falling directly on the page. The next best method would be in bright daylight without direct sun. And the least ideal way would be indoors with strong light, which should still work.

Take out the "Large and Small Print" page. Read the normal size print at a normal distance, where the letters are clear but not crisp, and not completely comfortable to read. You might not be able to make out a letter or two, or perhaps even a word or two, but you should be able to read most of it. Do not strain; just look at the letters. Make sure to blink and wave one hand around your periphery to ensure that you don't strain. When you look at the letters that are fuzzy, don't be upset. Allow them to be fuzzy. As you wave your hands quickly to the side, in 50 percent of all cases, they become slightly clearer because it allows more parts of the brain to start working, including the periphery. This will also help you to see well because it encourages the brain to notice more of the periphery and not to overstrain your central vision.

Next, obstruct your strong eye with a small piece of black paper, two inches by two inches, and look at the very, very large print. Bring the page all the way to your face until the page is almost touching your eyelashes, closer than the tip of your nose. Read the print, letter by letter, or part of each letter, point by point, reading aloud and waving your hand so you can see it in the periphery of the obstructed strong eye. Instead of moving your eyes the way you would when you normally read, you will move the paper so that each letter falls right in front of your eye, in your focal point. Wave your hand quickly in the periphery to take the strain off reading so close. Do this for two minutes.

Now hold the paper back eighteen inches, and read the normal print again. This is an induced stress on the eye rather than one of which we are unaware, and it strains the eye. Nevertheless, this will strengthen the ciliary muscle. In 80 percent of my clients and students, this works both momentarily and, with continued practice, long term,

You can do the same exercise with the shifter, although the letters are more important. Using the shifter twice a week can help you, in a neutral way, to move your weaker eye up and down and force the ciliary muscles of that eye—and reflexively, the ones of the strong eye—to start working better and become stronger. The lens then becomes more convex and more flexible.

Extra Exercise 5 for Presbyopia: Unfreezing

It is amazing how much our patterns control us. If you tend not to move much because you watch television a lot, sit at a computer all day, or drive for a living, it can eventually lead to a frozen back, a frozen gaze, frozen looks, and quite often, repetitive thoughts in your brain. Even if you are intellectually advanced, you may freeze the way in which you look and the way in which you move.

If you are a long-distance runner, you may run with a constant sense of freeze, meaning that you tighten your shoulders, neck, chest, and lower back when you run. Or if you lift weights, you may tense every part of your body in order to lift them. So, a sense of freeze may be the starting point from which you function.

One of the most important things for you to learn is how to unfreeze yourself. Regardless of what your lifestyle is, you could be frozen.

If your lifestyle is one of sitting, it's important for you to be comfortable when you sit, not just to *think* that you're comfortable. You should be properly supported in your seat so that you do not damage your back and neck from freezing your posture. It's likewise important to know that your eyes are relaxed, not frozen. How do you know that your eyes are relaxed? Simple: first of all, they blink; second, you have a sense of periphery when you look straight ahead.

Eye exercises are the beginning of unfreezing. Body movement is also the beginning of unfreezing. Unfreezing is more than a thing to do; it is a philosophy that you share.

It is so important to improve your presbyopia because it is one of the best preventions against cataracts. Cataracts happen because we don't take care of presbyopia. We allow the lens to be stiff, the ciliary muscles of the lens to be weak, and the lens then becomes more frozen, eventually leading to cellular change, and cataracts may appear. Remember that looking at a distance is one of the best exercises we do to negate the fact that life forces us to look from close up so much, as in reading and looking at computers and at cell phones.

It is crucial for us to allow the lens to be as flexible as possible and to not allow the presbyopia to increase in numbers all the time. Just like physicians tell you that in your forties it's normal to have presbyopia, they will tell you that in your sixties it's normal to have cataracts. But that is not true. Cataracts, unlike the one I was born with, are the result of our lifestyles and of looking close up, especially at pixels. This is because they are fuzzy at the margins but only clear at the center, which becomes an eyestrain. The result is basically a frozen lens, and just like a frozen joint that is not moving well leads to arthritis, a frozen lens could lead to cataracts. We really suggest that you mobilize, guard, and value your lens so it will not decay. Removing it is easy for competent medical specialists. But maintaining it takes work.

Correcting Astigmatism

Astigmatism is caused by an irregularly shaped cornea or an irregularly shaped lens. It is difficult to describe what the world looks like to people who experience astigmatism. Oftentimes, people with astigmatism have the sense that they see several images of objects at once. For example, when they look at the moon they may see the image of a clear moon along with a shadow moon, two shadow moons, or several shadow moons side by side. Even if they close one eye, they may still see more than one moon.

Often astigmatism accompanies nearsightedness or farsightedness. So a progressive way of improving your eyes would be to simultaneously work on correcting the myopia, hyperopia, and presbyopia while also addressing the astigmatism.

After practicing the recommended exercise program for astigmatism for two months, the astigmatism may disappear. It is then advisable to return to these exercises for one week every six months, for several years, in order to prevent the astigmatism from recurring.

Note for Astigmatic Readers

Beyond your program, you must do extra looking into the distance, extra palming, and also extra sunning throughout your day. What happens is that even though you do the program, when you sit at your computer again for four hours or so, you are going to decrease the benefit you have gained with these exercises. By regularly looking into the distance and palming, you give your eyes the opportunity to rest and to maintain more of the progress you have made with your vision.

Therefore, you must take moments throughout your day to add to your program. If you have been looking closely at your computer screen for an hour, take some time and look into the distance. Palm two or three times a day, for no less than six minutes each time, but don't forget to blink, and to breathe freely and deeply.

Exercise Program for Astigmatism

Sunning: 10 minutes daily.
Palming: 45 minutes minimum, 6 minutes at a time.
Headlines: 20 minutes daily.
Glow in the Dark: 20 minutes daily.

Extra Exercise 1 for Astigmatism: Headlines

Note: If you are farsighted, this is a great exercise to practice before starting to work on your other exercises.

For this exercise, you will need an eye chart taped to the wall at eye level, your cheap sunglasses with the lens popped out of the side for the eye that is weaker from a distance and the lens on the strong eye's side covered with opaque tape, and a large newspaper headline or large print from the Large and Small Print page.

Stand at a distance from the eye chart so that you can see the top third of the chart clearly without much straining, but you have to strain to see the bottom two-

Figure 4.7. Headlines exercise for astigmatism.

thirds. Basically, you are going to look at the eye chart while quickly waving the headlines in front of your face. Look past the blur of the headlines being waved in your face, and try to read the eye chart. Every few seconds, stop waving the headlines and look quickly at them. Blurt out the first letter you see clearly. Now wave the page again back and forth, and go back to reading the eye chart. The object is to quickly shift your focus from far to near, and back to far again.

If you have a partner with whom to practice these exercises, you can do this exercise a little differently. While you are reading the eye chart, your partner can very quickly flash fingers in front of your face, very close to your eyes, and you can tell your partner how many fingers they are holding up. Of course, this way is not good if you are by yourself because you cannot surprise yourself with your own fingers.

Figure 4.8. Variation on the headlines exercise for astigmatism.

So when you are practicing by yourself, pick up the page with the large headline and quickly wave it back and forth in front of your eyes, while looking at the chart. Read the chart aloud even if all you can read is the first three lines; do so repeatedly. Now, for less than half a second, stop waving the headlines, look at the large print, and say the first letter you can see. If you are in a phase of half guessing and half seeing because of the speed, that's exactly where you want you to be. Then return to waving the page back and forth.

Let's say that you are reading the letters on the top line of the eye chart. As you wave the piece of paper with the headline back and forth in front of your face very quickly, you might see the words "moving economy" in your periphery. What you want to do is to wave the paper so quickly that when you stop you may only see 'e'; then you keep waving it and say the letter *e* as you return your gaze to the chart and read the top line of letters once again. Then you stop waving the paper, and you may see the letter *c* or the letter *o*. Announce it aloud; then wave the paper and read the top line of the chart again. It is good to speak with a loud voice as you do these eye exercises, so that you distract yourself from focusing on the exercise itself. This will make it much more effective.

The next phase is to improve your near vision by trying this same exercise with the page of big and small print in front of you instead of an eye chart. This way you are working on the eye chart from afar and the page with big and small print from nearby.

Now put on your cheap sunglasses, with the lens removed on the side you look through with your weak eye and the lens of the glass in front of the strong eye covered with opaque tape. Again, wave the paper with the large print in front of your weaker eye while looking at the chart. Read the top line of the chart aloud while waving the headline back and forth in front of your face. From time to time, stop waving the headlines in front of your face for half a second, enough time to guess a letter that you see. After ten times doing this, look at the chart with your weak eye, but without waving the headline in the air. You may be able to clearly read an extra line on the chart. Then take off the glasses, and you may be able to clearly read two extra lines on the chart.

So when we do this exercise for astigmatism, we don't try to look at small print but instead look at large print on the chart from far away and near, and at regular size print—like this book—from a regular distance, or even from far away when it's easier for us to see the print. The point is not to look at something small but to look at something large with a greater ease. When the brain stops you from having the astigmatism, the astigmatism just slowly disappears because the eye finds the mechanism to do it with. One working theory that hasn't been proven yet is the ciliary muscles create a pool of liquid in front of them and on the cornea, which slowly straightens the cornea and flattens it, and therefore brings it back to its spherical shape.

Extra Exercise 2 for Astigmatism: Glow in the Dark

Note: We do this exercise because we want the eye to move around. We have found, in our experience, that many people have an easier time moving their eyes in a rotating motion in the dark.

The idea is to follow the glowing objects with your eye, and not by moving your whole head. Move your eyes only, so that your eye muscles are stretching. The stretching motion changes the structure of the eyes with time. People say the cornea cannot change shape, but they are wrong.

For this exercise, you will need a glow-in-the-dark ball, a dark room, and a strip of paper to tape to your nose. The paper should stretch from the top of your forehead to the bottom of your chin, the same as in the Melissa Exercise mentioned previously in this book and also in the next chapter on cross-sightedness.

Eventually, this exercise gets simple, but it's difficult to master at first. All you do is tape the paper from your forehead to your chin so that it covers your whole nose and obstructs the first third of each eye. Turn the lights off in your room, and play catch with the glow-in-the-dark ball. Throw the ball from hand to hand above your head so that the ball crosses the visual plane in front of your face. It should disappear briefly as it passes the paper taped to your head. You can also practice bouncing the ball off the wall, throwing it with one hand and catching it with the other. Remember not to move your whole head to track the location of the ball. Only move your eyeballs, so that they can stretch to their full range of motion in both directions.

Imagine doing curls with your biceps, but only bending your arms a little bit. You would not be getting the full benefit of the exercise, and you may even damage the very part of your body you are attempting to build up. Just like the curl of the biceps or lifting weights with partial tension, we don't move the eyes fully and put great pressure only on part of the extrinsic eye muscles. This idea is the same when it comes to your eyes. Exercise the eye muscles by watching the glowing ball in the dark, and moving your eyes the full range of their possible motion; this will stretch, and even change, the shape of your cornea over time.

Chapter 5

Overcoming Cross-Sightedness and Lazy Eye

Correcting Cross-Sightedness

Amblyopia and strabismus are both terms for cross-sightedness, and they have something in common. They both refer to a "lazy eye," but with amblyopia the eyes do not look cross-sighted to an outside observer. With strabismus, however, the eyes actually look crossed. I have heard people sometimes joke that strabismus is when one eye is so beautiful that the other eye just wants to look at it all the time. It is okay to have a sense of humor. And this really is true: every part of you is beautiful, even your strabismus. With amblyopia and strabismus, the brain shuts off the information coming from one eye, but only in strabismus do the eyes look crossed to the outside observer. And the term "lazy eye" is actually a misnomer. In reality, the brain is just not using one of the eyes.

If you have cross-sightedness, you have two problems. The first is that your brain favors one eye over the other and works that eye while it suppresses the other eye from working at all or nearly as much as it needs to. This is why some people refer to cross-sighted people as having a "lazy eye."

The other problem with strabismus, or amblyopia, is that doctors do not believe you can improve your condition in any way. Doctors mistakenly believe that, after the age of eight, cross-sighted people can no longer learn how to get their two eyes to work together. The debate over the plasticity or elasticity of the brain is ongoing, but old concepts are giving way to new understandings. More and more people understand that the brain can change if it's being exercised properly.

As I mentioned earlier, the oldest person I've worked with so far was 101 years old. He experienced great changes from his exercises, and he was able to see better and to improve his brain and eye function significantly. I have also worked with several elderly patients, some in their eighties and nineties, and have witnessed positive changes in their visual systems. There is no doubt in my mind that no matter what age you are, you can change the function of your eyes; there is enough elasticity in your brain to back it up.

The issue isn't age, but whether or not a person is practicing the correct exercises for his or her age. It may work easier for a five-year-old child to put on a patch for four or eight hours a day as he or she plays, in order to get used to the weaker eye working. Indeed, the brain has more plasticity when you're five than when you're seventy-five. But, there are good, age-appropriate exercises you can do at any age that can change your visual system completely.

In addition to the exercises in this section, it is essential to do some of the previously mentioned exercises as well, including the ten steps in chapter 2. Especially helpful for cross-sightedness is the exercise in the section on astigmatism called "Glow in the Dark." As I mentioned in the introduction to chapter 4, it is important to refer back to that chapter for an extensive explanation of the exercises I recommend in this section. In addition to extensively describing the exercise steps, there is important information regarding the benefits of these recommended practices.

One other wonderful practice for you is to lie down twice a day, with a warm towel over your closed eyes. One of the recommendations that I normally make is to soak the towel in warm herbal tea. Do not use boiling water, just warm water. Within two or three minutes, the towel tends to cool off then you want to put a cold towel that has been placed wet in the freezer for two minutes or in the refrigerator for fifteen minutes and keep it over your closed eyes for a minute or two. You will find that the eyes are much more relaxed. That pleasant feeling can improve your circulation and increase your level of relaxation when you start to work for further improvement. The reason to do this with the towels is to alleviate the strain you have caused your eyes after doing the other exercises. Relaxation must be something you prioritize after doing all of them. Alleviate the strain with a wet towel.

Also, and this is especially vital for cross-sightedness, make sure you are practicing breathing exercises daily, and receiving face, neck, and back massages from a very good massage therapist at least once a month, but preferably much more often.

Exercise Program for Cross-Sightedness:
At Least 90 Minutes a Day

Sunning: 10 minutes daily.
Palming: 12 minutes daily.
Long Swing: 10 minutes daily.
Glow in the Dark: 10 minutes daily.
Walking Backward: 5 minutes daily.
Blink Each Eye Independently: 5 minutes daily.
Extra Exercise for Cross-Sightedness: 30 minutes daily.

Note: I cannot stress enough how important it is to make these exercises a regular part of your daily routine. Whatever you are doing, you can also practice your eye exercises. While you are waiting for a bus, you can do your sunning. While you are riding the bus, you can look far into the distance. You can always be looking at details. At work, instead of taking cigarette or coffee breaks, take breaks to practice long swinging or palming. Anywhere there is a dark room, you can practice throwing a glow-in-the-dark ball around. Don't just practice for one hour or two hours at home. Incorporate these exercises into every aspect of your life. That is the way to give yourself good vision for life.

For your extra daily exercise, you may choose from any of the following. The main point with cross-sightedness is to train the brain to use both eyes, not to favor one eye over the other. All of the following extra exercises do just that.

Extra Exercises for Cross-Sightedness: Rotate the Eyes;
Look into the Darkness

Sit in a dark room, looking straight ahead. Sit up and don't lie down for this exercise. Now move your eyes in a rotating motion in the dark. Within a few minutes, even a dark room seems to have some light. Move your eyes from area to area in the dark room. Look up, and move the eyes from side to side in the room; then look down, and move your eyes from side to side while the eyes are looking down. Now close one eye and slowly move the full range of rotation with the open eye: up, to the side, and down. Then switch which eye is closed, and repeat.

The next exercise you can do in the dark, or not. Palm, but not real palming; just do it for three breaths. Take your hand off of the amblyopic or strabismus eye while covering the stronger eye and look at your thumb, while moving it in a wide rotation. Even in the dark you can see at least the dark form of your thumb. Move your thumb in full rotating motion, in both directions, as you follow it. Now switch and do exactly the same with your other eye. We do this to stretch the external muscles that, to some extent, are responsible for the cross-sightedness.

Mirror Images

Next is a mirror exercise. If your left eye is the one that turns in, look in the mirror while covering the right eye. Normally, when you cover the right eye, the left eye should be totally straight because the two retinas and the two eyes are not competing; but sometimes it isn't. In this case, tilt your head a bit to the right and look intensively at the left side, and let the left eye be straighter. Do it several times and palm for thirty seconds to relax your eyes.

Now look at the bridge of your nose. Do not look at the right eye; do not look at the left eye. Look at the bridge of your nose between both eyes, and you will see both eyes. If they tend to cross, this is exactly what your brain will correct automatically. For your brain, normally, is not as aware of the cross-sightedness as you may think. You may see it in pictures. You may even sense it from time to time. But when you face the mirror and you look in between your eyes, so your central vision is on the bridge of your nose and your peripheral vision is from both sides, you can exactly see the cross-sightedness. It's amazing how much the brain tends to correct what appears to be wrong, and the cross-sightedness can decrease. If the eye tends to tremor a bit, the tremor will stop.

In addition to this exercise, as you stand in front of the mirror, move your hips in a rotating motion. Don't stop looking in the mirror while your hips are moving. That helps to distract you, but it also helps you to get more circulation to your eyes. If the hips are loose, the ribs will be looser, and your breathing will get deeper. Your neck will get loose as well, and more blood will flow to your eyes.

Quite often, the shortening of one muscle, versus the lengthening of its opponent, has to do with poor blood flow to that muscle. So, remember to look in the mirror often while moving your hips in a rotating motion. If your vision is good, you can do this in any light. In fact, dim light may be the best light you can do it in, because it rests the eyes. If your vision is poor, you must have strong light that will show you your face in the mirror.

By now you know that anytime there is an indication of effort in doing this exercise or any other, you must palm. Palming is going to help you to reduce the stress and to renew the work. Also, you can look into the distance before doing the Mirror Exercise.

I found that my Mirror Exercise was one of the best exercises to reduce my strabismus. You see, I struggled with strabismus from a very young age. In fact, in my case, the eyes never communicated because I was blind around the time that most people have their eyes working together, which is between four and six months of age. Since I was blind during that time, my brain had never developed straight eyes. In 1992, at the age of thirty-eight, I received my passport picture, and my eyes were severely cross-sighted. Six months before the expiration of that passport, the Brazilian Consulate issued me a five-year visa stamped on that passport. New pictures were taken in 2002, when I was forty-eight, so I had two passports to compare. I took these passports to my school. Before going to the Brazilian Consulate to verify that I could use both passports, my good colleague and student looked at the passport pictures and said, "My goodness, look how your eyes have improved!" My cross-sightedness (strabismus) had decreased, and my eyes straightened by 75 percent in ten years. Since then, I laugh at the fact that I lost hair and grew older by ten years, and yet my eyes got straighter. At the age of fifty-seven, I had to take another picture before going to Brazil for the Brazilian visa. So, before taking the picture, I went to Mount Tamalpais—a beautiful mountain in Marin County in the San Francisco area—and looked at the whole Bay area, and looked into the distance, and it helped to straighten my eyes. It is a very dynamic process. At times my eyes cross a bit and at other times they straighten. Now, years later, my eyes are even straighter. And so, straightening your eyes is definitely possible in your forties and fifties, but it is also possible in your seventies and eighties. You just need to do the work. Now, in my sixties, my eyes only cross when they are fatigued, and are completely straight when they are relaxed.

Figure 5.1. Passport pictures taken ten years apart. My eyes had straightened by 75 percent.

Looking in a mirror was one of my main exercises. I used to stand in elevators if they had good light and, for a moment, look in a mirror at the bridge of my nose between both eyes. Often, however, people with cross-sightedness look far into the distance, and their cross-sightedness is decreased; sometimes it disappears. The reason is deep relaxation of the eyes.

The Melissa Exercise

The most wonderful exercise for cross-sightedness is the Melissa Exercise. Melissa was the director of my School for Self-Healing for ten years. These days, she is a great practitioner and teacher of Self-Healing in Texas, and was featured in the movie *Happy*. She was interviewed in this documentary because of her ability to be a very happy person despite having experienced great tragedy. She was in an accident in which her face, chest, and ribs were crushed by a Chevrolet Suburban. She had a great many surgeries to reconstruct her face. After one of these surgeries, her eye turned in and lost a lot of vision. She also saw double. She became interested in my work even before she had started extensive training and long individual sessions. The exercise of putting a small piece of paper on the bridge of her nose, then using a large piece of paper and waving to the side, was useful, but she saw double below and above it. So I simply devised a piece of paper that I would place on her nose so that it stretched from her forehead to her chin. I put masking tape on the top and bottom, and had her throw a ball from hand to hand above her head. She could see the ball with each eye, and her vision was not double for a while; this provided great relief for her visual system as well as her neck, for her neck

hurt constantly due to the uneven-
ness of her eyes.

This is a great exercise to help
people with cross-sightedness. If
you put a piece of paper between
your eyes and throw a ball from
side to side, at least one hundred
times for about two minutes, the
ball will disappear for a split second—because of its speed you will
not notice it—before you see the
ball again with the other eye. That
will create a very nice difference in
your eyes. The dominant eye will
no longer control the eye that trails.

Figure 5.2. As you do the Melissa Exercise, the
brain will use both eyes independently.

To a great extent, that's the
essence of all amblyopia and stra-
bismus: a lazy eye. And a lazy eye is not lazy on its own. Often, it's an
eye that doesn't see well. Sometimes, however, it's an eye that sees very
well, but the brain is not using it. The brain did not learn to use both eyes
together, and so, throughout your life, one eye looked and the other one
trailed. Until now, the brain did not learn to use both eyes together; it used
only the strong or dominant eye. As you do this exercise, the brain will
use both eyes independently.

With this division between the two eyes, each eye looks and sees the ball
independently. The right eye will see the ball in the right hand; the left eye
will see the ball in the left hand. There is a body-eye connection here that
makes it very real for the body and the eyes. This is not a peripheral exercise. In fact, look at the ball. When you throw the ball from the right to the
left or the left to the right, there is a moment when you do not see the ball
as you throw it above your head. That's good because, in a brief moment,
you will see the ball and your hand will have to respond to what you see.
Eye-hand coordination is very precious in this case because it makes it real
to your brain that you are actually using the lazy eye, as well as the eye
you always use. It's not our purpose to use the lazy eye more than the eye

that is always used. Our purpose in this exercise is to use both of them.

The use of both eyes may give you great relief. If it is hard for you to do a hundred repetitions, then start with ten, and palm after taking the paper off. If it's easy, continue to do it three or four times a day. And, if that's easy, then do it for ten minutes, three times a day for a month. You will feel much looser and your muscles will work much better. This happens for two reasons: one, because each eye works independently, which is a big, important first step; two, because each eye looks down and up to follow the ball.

Clap

Next, throw the ball from hand to hand above your head with the piece of paper, and clap your hands before you catch the ball. That will really distract you, and will also activate you in a way that will have your brain building new pathways to be able to see with the weaker eye.

So, for example, if your left eye is your weaker eye and you clap your hands before you catch the ball with one hand, it's going to be easier for you to catch the ball on the right side than on the left side. With enough practice, however, it's going to be easy to catch on both sides, and it's going to start to be natural for you to see with your weaker eye.

Walk

Next is to walk as you throw the ball from hand to hand above your head while doing the Melissa Exercise. Walk forward while throwing the ball from hand to hand above your head. Walk backward. Walk sideways. It should become more and more challenging, but also more and more relaxing for your eyes.

Jump

Now try to jump when you throw the ball from hand to hand above your head. Jump on the ground or, if you are able to, jump on a trampoline, which is the best method. You will see the periphery moving in the background, while wearing the Melissa paper on your face. You'll also be throwing the ball from hand to hand above your head and trying to catch it each time you bounce.

Combinations

Challenge yourself to combine all levels of the Melissa Exercise. Walk while throwing the ball from hand to hand above your head, and also clap your hands before you catch the ball. Walk backward and sideways while you combine clapping. Combine clapping with jumping or bouncing on the trampoline. Or, finally, the most difficult variation of the Melissa Exercise is to keep both eyes open, throw the ball up, and then close the eye that does not need to see the ball.

For example, with your two eyes open, throw the ball from the right hand to the left hand. As the ball reaches the area above your head, close your right eye, and with the left eye you will see the ball. Catch the ball with your left hand, and then open both eyes. Throw the ball above your head again and, as the ball reaches the area above your head where the two eyes cannot see, close your left eye and catch the ball with your right hand.

Do this for a while, then go back to the original Melissa Exercise. Perform the most basic variation, keeping your two eyes open, while throwing the ball above your head and catching it. See how much you have improved, and how simple this original method seems now that you have expanded your comfort zone and have adapted to your new challenges.

The Melissa Exercise is very important for cross-sightedness, and I recommend that you practice it often.

The "Melissinia" Exercise

Even for people who can see with two eyes, we recommend this variation of the Melissa Exercise because there needs to be a balance within each eye. The Melissinia Exercise was originally invented for people who see only with one eye; however, most people have weakness in one eye. What I recommend is to do it more with the eye that is weak but also to do it with the eye that is strong; in this way, you do it with both eyes. Whichever way you do it, it should be three times as much with the weaker eye. For example, you can do three minutes with the weak eye and 1 minute with the strong eye. It creates a new balance within each eye, which in turn helps to create a more balanced use within each eye.

Figure 5.3. Throw the ball from side to side above the head, just as you did in the Melissa Exercise.

So, first patch your strong eye, then put a very thin (one-eighth of an inch) but long enough strip of construction paper over your weaker eye, from your forehead to your cheekbone; its thinness will only cover a small part of your central vision. Now take a ball and throw it from hand to hand above your head. Next, take a strip of paper slightly thicker (one-quarter of an inch), and do the same. The third time, try it with a piece of paper slightly under three-eighths of an inch. And each time, throw the ball from side to side, just as you did in the Melissa Exercise, except this time using one eye. You can do the same patching in both eyes, but the recommended procedure is to do it much more on the weaker eye. Do it for five minutes at a time. The reason for this exercise is to allow more parts of the eye itself to be active. If one of your eyes sees well, more or less, and the other eye has areas of diminished sight—scotomas, which are blind spots—this would be a great exercise, providing your eye can see the ball; it is not relevant to old people. It should be done once a week at first, but eventually just once a month, to make sure each eye moves enough in a rotating motion.

The latest discovery of using the Melissa Exercise with a neurological patient makes me think that cross-sighted people could use the same approach from time to time. I still recommend the patch, but try also to use a Melissa, meaning the long strip of paper that you put on your nose earlier, but now put it over one eye. So while you're covering the eye, you're not patching it, but rather you're obstructing the central vision, the central peripheral vision, and some of the peripheral vision. Then do exactly the same Melissa Exercise we were talking about—the three different strips—with a ball. What happens, especially when you work on the weak eye, is that the strong eye has some light penetrating it and the brain is not getting as stretched. This is because you don't completely cover the strong eye and stop it from working, but you stop it from working around 80 to 90 percent, and so there is the realization in the brain that the strong eye is still doing something. Again, covering the weak eye with the Melissa and working with the Melissinia and the strong eye about a third or a quarter of the time that you work with the weak eye can also make a big difference.

Beads on a String

Your job in this exercise is to teach your brain what to focus on and what not to focus on. First, make a string of beads with five different colors of beads on it. At the School for Self-Healing, we have strings of beads you can use for this exercise. Tie one end of the string of beads to something in front of you, like the back of a chair or the railing of your patio. Now hold the string of beads in front of your eyes. Focus on the different colored beads. As you focus on each separate bead, every bead that you focus on must appear to be a single bead. Every bead that you don't focus on must appear to be doubled.

For example, if you have five beads, when you focus on the first bead, the second, third, fourth, and fifth beads should appear to be

Figure 5.4. Your job in this exercise is to teach your brain what to focus on and what not to focus on.

doubled. When you focus on the third, the first two and last two will look doubled, and the middle should look single. When you focus on the fifth bead, the first four will look doubled and the last one should look single.

What often happens to people with cross-sightedness is that, first of all, they may not see double with the beads that are in their periphery; they may see single beads all along. The best exercise to correct this is to look at one bead, let's say the closest one to you, and close your eyes one at a time. When you close your eyes one at a time, you can see a shift, a move of the beads from side to side. While doing this, keep thinking and focusing on the bead in front of you, with each eye separately. That means you keep looking at that bead, but you will see all the beads shifting angles, because each eye sees the bead from a different angle, and even from a different distance. Only when both eyes are open can your brain measure the distances more precisely. After doing it forty times, open both eyes, and when you look at the first bead, the rest should appear to be doubled.

The bead you are focusing on is being viewed with your central vision. The ones you are not directly looking at are being viewed with your peripheral vision. The nervous system and the brain see one image with central vision and two separate images with peripheral vision. So, even if you look at an object straight in front of you, but you focus on another object in front of *that* object, then the object you focus on will appear to be single, and the one you don't focus on will appear to be doubled. You want to become capable of distinguishing between the one you look at directly and the one that you don't, so that the one you are looking at appears to be single and the one you aren't looking at appears to be doubled.

Your goal is to be very relaxed when you look at one bead and see the rest doubled. Never strain to do that because that does not help anything. A way to not strain is to look into the distance either in the beginning or in the middle of the exercise, maybe wave your hands quickly to the side, and then return to the exercise. Another way is to move one of your hands: let's say the left one holds the strings at the bridge of your nose and so the right would move from right to left and left to right, thus providing you with a sense of periphery. Remember, when your two eyes are looking together, normally there is no sense of strain; therefore, looking into the distance and noticing your periphery are good ways not to strain the eyes. Even if you practice this for a few seconds at a time, you will start to relax your eyes almost completely. Then when you feel that your eyes are completely relaxed, extend the time that you look at the beads. Sometimes, this period can extend up to five minutes; longer sessions—or marathon sessions, as we call them—can last as long as ten minutes if you don't lose your patience. Remember, the purpose of this exercise is deep relaxation of the eyes through balanced use. If you strain in the process, stop and do another exercise.

Holding Double

If you were able to see double, the next point is to hold the double. You will find that most people who can produce a double image can hold it for thirty seconds, maybe even a whole minute, before they become fatigued. When this happens, of course, they should massage around their eyes, palm or sun, look into the distance, or do long swinging until the fatigue goes away. You can blink as you do the exercise and, hopefully, you won't lose the double image.

Your goal is to be able to hold a double for ten slow breaths. You can move from one double to another. You can see the front bead as single and all the other four as doubles. You can move through the five beads, one after another, and hold each double for ten breaths. So you don't have to stay at one point for the full ten breaths, but you should continuously see double for the duration.

As long as the strain is not too high, this is a great exercise for good coordination between the two eyes. Sometimes you will have only thirty seconds and sometimes you can have as much as seven or eight minutes in which to do it; either way, you should do it as many times as possible each day. Doing this once a day for ten breaths per bead will make a big difference. If your eyes do not get tired from seeing double, it is a very good indication of relaxation and a good use of the two eyes. On the other hand, if they get tired for any reason, you can look into the distance and then look back at the beads, or move your hand from side to side, from right to left and left to right, all the way in your periphery. When the two peripheries work, there could never be fatigue. Similarly, when the two centers work in unison and one does not suppress the other, or at least doesn't suppress it much, there can never be fatigue. These two things are parallel and work together, which is why you want to repeat this exercise many times. In fact, it's sometimes beneficial to do a marathon session for a longer time that you breathe. For example, up to seven or eight minutes at a time of looking at doubles will make a huge difference.

Two-Color Exercise (Beak Glasses)

This exercise uses a tool we sometimes refer to in fun as "beak glasses." We call them beak glasses because they are glasses with two strips of paper attached to the front of them in such a way that they stick straight out between the lenses. When you put them on, it looks as if you were wearing a two-colored beak.

The pieces of paper should be two different colors; for example, one could be orange and the other could be yellow. Put on the glasses and look straight ahead into the distance. Now toss a tennis ball from one hand to the other and try to catch the ball. Toss the ball several times.

Since the paper is attached to the front of the glasses, you are guaranteed to be using both of your eyes for this exercise. When the ball is on the left side of your body, it emphasizes to the left eye that the left color exists. When the

Figure 5.5. "Beak glasses." When the ball is on the right side, it emphasizes to the right eye that the right color exists.

ball is on the right side, it emphasizes to the right eye that the right color exists. As the ball travels from side to side above the head, the peripheral vision of both eyes is being worked individually; the central vision is still looking straight ahead into the distance. Remember that the central vision sees a mostly still picture, while the peripheral vision sees movement.

One interesting thing about this exercise is to notice which color each eye seems to be seeing. If your eyes are completely at ease and completely functional, when you look into the distance you will see the two colors, each one of them on the opposite side. And this will indicate that they work well together.

If one of these colors disappears, you can also quickly wave your hand close to your eye; not so close that it's dangerous, but right in front of the eye. Often, that color will reappear. Seeing two colors with both eyes, especially for someone who has a hard time using both eyes together, could be a very relaxing experience at certain times.

Besides the glasses with the two colors, we also have a little stick with two colors, which we put on the bridge of the nose as we look into the distance. We don't look at the two colors, *we see them*. So we look into the distance while seeing those two colors at the same time, which, like seeing double at the same time, indicates deep relaxation and that the two eyes are working together. Moreover, being able to rest your eyes at a distance and from near, and to move relatively quickly—less than thirty seconds, from near to far—also indicates eye relaxation. Remember, amblyopia and strabismus are conditions for which relaxation rarely exists, and achieving it could help your life in many ways. And this also goes for people without amblyopia and strabismus. We all need these exercises because we make our eyes rigid throughout our life, and we need to reduce that rigidity all we can.

Figure 5.6. A little stick with two colors, which we put on the bridge of the nose as we look into the distance.

Red and Green Glasses

Each color has different wavelengths. For example, the color red has long wavelengths and the color green has short wavelengths. If you look through a pair of glasses with one green lens and one red lens, quite often the colors of the objects you look at seem to be different through the red lens than through the green. Some colors you can see more easily with the red, and others you can see more easily with the green.

Figure 5.7. Working with red and green glasses made it possible for me to have partial three-dimensional vision.

When you look at the world with both eyes through the red-and-green filter, you will see quite a few amazing things. For example, if you walk in a park or in your garden with red-and-green glasses on, you're going to find that you see a pinkish view of flowers through the red lens but, at the same time, you see a greenish view of leaves much clearer with your green lens. So, from time to time, close one eye and look at colors with the open eye; then close that eye and open the other, and see what colors you notice. Do the pink flower petals disappear when you close the eye looking through the red lens? Do the green leaves disappear when you look only through the red lens? Now look around. Take a few minutes to enjoy three-dimensional vision with both eyes open.

You'll find, however, that if you close the eye looking through the red lens and you look at the pink or reddish flower only through the green lens, it will not look red or pink to you; rather, it will look dark, which is far from its true color. If you close the eye looking through the green lens and look only through the red, the green leaves would look dark.

In fact, this is exactly how you start to develop bilateral vision and three-dimensional vision. You emphasize to yourself the difference between the two eyes. Your two eyes are independent. No one eye sees what the other one sees; therefore, no one eye controls the other. Instead, each is independent of the other, and the brain fuses the image equally from both of them.

In the past, I had no three-dimensional vision. I didn't know if an object was close to me or far away from me. But as I improved my acuity and could see large freeway signs, I wanted to be able to drive. Working with red and green glasses made it possible for me to have partial three-dimensional vision, and to eventually see well enough to start learning to drive and to know where I was on the road.

In your case, you may not have such a dramatic change, but having better three-dimensional vision and having a distinction between the two eyes is a great way to reduce your cross-sightedness.

Object and Line

The first step is to make a division between the two eyes completely and to unite them in the brain. Wearing the red-and-green glasses, you'll see light with one eye and an object with the other eye. Or some people will not see light or an object. The aim of this exercise is to get both eyes working together.

For this exercise you will need a red pen or pencil, a piece of white paper, and a small flashlight with a red bulb. If you don't have a red bulb, put some red duct tape or two layers of red cellophane paper glued with masking tape over the flashlight lens to simulate a red filter.

Draw a red circle on the white sheet of paper. Hold the paper out in front of you with one hand, so that the paper is parallel to the ground, about a foot in front of your eyes. Turn the flashlight on and put it underneath the paper, making sure the flashlight is touching the paper and shining the light up through it. Look down at the circle while shining the light up through the paper. You should see the circle and also the light.

It's very important to put the red over your weaker eye because the brain is much more attracted to light than to form. The circle or lines—vertical, horizontal—would all be forms, and the brain is much more interested in light. Similarly, if you are walking down the street and you see a light in a shop, you would find that your eyes are much more attracted to that shop than to a shop without one.

Now close your red-filtered eye. The eye that looks through the green filter should see the circle but not the light, because the red light cannot penetrate through the green lens. On the other hand, the green filter does not stop you from seeing the red circle.

Conversely, if you close the eye that looks through the green, and only look through the red lens, you will see the light, but you will not see the red circle. The eye with the green filter will only see the object, and the eye with the red filter will only see the light. This kind of division is very important because you see a separate image from the eye with the red filter and the eye with the green filter simultaneously.

Now move the light, which is underneath the page, around the perimeter of the circle, like you are tracing around its edge. If your eyes can track together, you will be able to keep the light on the edge of the circle. If your eyes cannot track together, though you may think that the light is on the edge of the circle, it will actually be elsewhere. In my case, when I thought that the light was on the circle, the light was actually outside or inside the circle. So, a way for you to know what's happening with your light is to suddenly close the eye with the green filter; when you do this, you will see exactly where the light is. When you open the eye with the green filter, you will see if the light remains exactly where it was when that eye was closed, or if it moved. Even if it moved, don't correct it. Close your eyes and open them, ten to twenty times, until both eyes see the light exactly where it really is. Once it stays in the same place, it means that your eyes are tracking. It doesn't matter if it's in the circle or out; what matters is that the two eyes are looking together at the same spot.

You may find yourself in the middle of this exercise needing to palm. Palm for as long as you need to help you relax enough to return to the exercise.

Now change the glasses. That is, if you first put the red lens on the left eye and the green on the right eye, now put the green on the left eye and the red on the right eye; then repeat the exercise.

Figure 5.8. Turn the red flashlight on and put it underneath the paper, touching the paper, shining the light up through it.

One of the ways for you to know whether the light is in the circle is to ask someone else to let you know, because people who have strabismus or amblyopia do not often know on their own where the light is. They may think it's in the circle but it may be out of it. Another way is to raise your head up and look underneath the frame of the glasses, and then you'll know if the light is in the circle.

What I found is that many people are very upset when the light was not where they thought it was, and that is the biggest hurdle we have to work with—because now you have a good indicator that shows you if your eyes are working together. And if they don't work together, this is a good way for you to start getting them to work together. You may need to do many other exercises, like the Melissa Exercise—putting a long piece of paper between the eyes—and the relaxation exercises that we have mentioned for that to finally work. So it is worth your while to allow yourself not to do it right and to simply correct where you are. Doing these exercises is a way of slowly knowing where the light is in relation to the circle, since some kinds of vision make it difficult to distinguish its location.

Another exercise you can do with the red-and-green glasses is to have someone draw a line with the red pencil, and you try to trace the line while wearing the red filter over your strong eye. The reason for this is that through the red lens you will not be able to see red lines or red writing *unless* you are in the 2 percent of the population who can see a red line or red writing through a red lens. In that case, the other exercises are applicable to you, but not this one.

You want to put the red lens in front of the strong eye so the weaker eye will read the red print, but the stronger eye will not read the red line or print. The two eyes will see most other colors together, but the eye with the red filter won't be able to see whatever is red, and that changes domination for a moment, which could be five to eight minutes. The weaker eye will take a front seat and, as a result, the brain will learn to use it more in day-to-day activity.

The fact that you favor your weaker eye at this moment doesn't mean it doesn't stay weaker, but it means that you use it more now. And, it will participate more in the vision of both eyes. Just like it's easier to stand on two legs rather than one, it's easier to use both eyes rather than suppress one and use the other much more. So, the one that's being suppressed becomes very weak, the one that's always being worked becomes very tired, and in time, both become weak.

You can also draw a vertical line and a horizontal line; they can be pretty long, and you should be able follow them visually, with a red flashlight shining from underneath, touching the page with the flashlight. Some people can follow a horizontal line but not a vertical one; I had that problem. I could easily follow a horizontal line with both eyes tracing it, but I could not easily follow a vertical line. Some people find just the opposite. So whatever your challenge is, keep practicing. You may find that when the red lens is over your strong eye, you follow the line better, and when the red lens is over your weaker eye, you don't follow it as well. Again, the reason for this is that the brain is more attracted to light than to form. But it's important for you to do it from a neutral state. Don't do it for very long, but just for about three to four minutes at a time, every other day, until it becomes easy for you to do it. In some cases that I have seen, the light disappears when you try to trace a circle or a line. All you need to do is close your strong eye and the light will reappear immediately. But when you open it, it may disappear again. So open and close you strong eye ten times. You can also knock on the paper with the flashlight, or put the paper on a red translucent clipboard and knock with the flashlight on the clipboard. Many people then start to see the light and the circle or the lines at the same time. Some people have such poor fusion of the eyes that they will see the location of the light in one place and the location of the circle or the lines in another place. So that is their starting point. As you exercise, you can also draw line forms that you find are useful or helpful. Whether or not you do it right or wrong at first, with time, when you trace better, you'll find that your eyes are much straighter.

It's also really good to sit in daylight or in the sun and read red print. See the red chart in the back of the book. It's easy for you to create a red hardcopy of this book, for example, in different print sizes from your own computer and then to read it. One of our clients was bored with the red print that she had to read in English with the weaker eye. So we printed a French version of the story of *The Little Prince* in red because she was familiar with the French language—although it was a second language to her—which piqued her interest. The more you read with your weaker eye while the stronger eye is being blocked by the red color, the better it is.

It's also useful for you to draw and to write letters with a red pencil, and then to write them from the opposite end. So, for example, you write from left to right through a whole page (names of people and animals that you like or anything else), and then you write from bottom to top over the same letters that you have written from right to left. If you speak Hebrew, however, which is written right to left, you would do the opposite. Regardless, it's very important that you sit in strong light, which makes a big difference. In our school we have a balcony, and we take a folding table outside so that people can see the red line through the green lens with the help of the bright light of the outdoors. Again, it's also important that you know you're not straining or stressing. From time to time, you can even lie down and put a cold towel over your eyes to make sure there is no inflammation or stress in them.

Card Game

This is a fun and effective way to help balance the two eyes because you don't even realize that you're doing an exercise, and you create body-eye coordination as well. Let's say the left eye is weaker; it will now have to work no less than the right eye, which has no control over it in this situation.

You start off with a special deck of cards (two decks, if you have a few people playing) specifically designed to work with the red and green glasses. The deck is made up of two differently colored cards: half the deck is red with black letters, and the other half is white with red letters. You can only see the white cards with the green lens and the red cards with the red lens. As this game proceeds, you and others wear the glasses while you each simultaneously throw down a card from your own portion of the deck. When you identify certain numbers, you will react with a corresponding physical response. For instance, when you see a card with a nine on it, you clap your hands; when you see a seven, you tap your forehead; when you see an ace, you stamp on the floor and bang on the table, and so

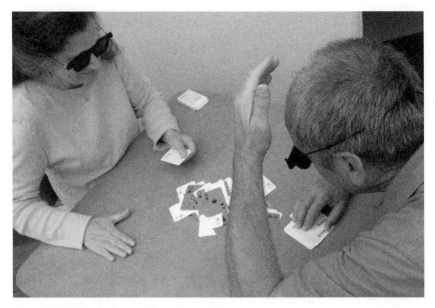

Figure 5.9. Playing a variation of the card game War.

on. The responses can match whatever four cards you would like them to match, and can be anything you are able to dream up. The point is to do something with your body in response to the numbers you have designated in the cards. The person who reacts the quickest when one of these cards is thrown is the one who gets to keep the pile. When it appears that about half of the cards have been thrown, reverse your glasses so that each eye has a chance to see through both the red filter and the green filter.

It's better, and more fun, to have two or three people playing this game along with you. Extra pairs of glasses are inexpensive and can be purchased at the School for Self-Healing, as can the cards themselves. As enjoyable as it is, this game has had significant results: there has been a temporary improvement in the vision of 50 percent of the people who have played it.

Nystagmus

Nystagmus is an involuntary flutter, a fast uncontrollable movement of the eyes that may happen in many different ways: up and down (vertical nystagmus), from side to side (horizontal nystagmus), or in rotation (rotary or torsional nystagmus). Depending on the cause, these movements may be in both eyes or in just one eye, but may result in limited vision due to the inability to focus on what one is looking at. Nystagmus may be caused by congenital disorders (including albinism—lack of pigment—and cataracts that were not operated on in time), acquired or central nervous system disorders, toxicity, pharmaceutical drugs, alcohol, or rotational movement.

There are ways to overcome nystagmus regardless of whether it is the result of cataract surgery, because of albinism, or for any other reason. You can do lots of palming every day, lie in dark rooms often, and do all ten steps of the vision exercises. After about two months of doing the ten steps, look in the mirror at the bridge of your nose between your two eyes, as described in the section on cross-sightedness. You will be able to see both eyes in your peripheral vision and you will sense the tremor in them. They will slow down simply because you see them in the mirror. When the brain senses a deficit, it tends to correct it automatically. It's a wonderful thing to experience. I've done it many times and it slowed down my nystagmus considerably: it used to be three hundred movements per minute, and now it's between zero and twelve.

When you look between the eyes, it's the best indicator that the eyes are moving. In response, the brain will immediately slow down the movement of the eyes. When you look between the two eyes, they are in the periphery, so your focus must be on the bridge of your nose or a small point on the bridge of your nose if your vision is acute. My vision was very poor, so looking between the eyes at the bridge of my nose from very near made that area seem big for me. Rarely did I find a patient who had nystagmus and still had perfect vision. Most of the time, nystagmus is an indication of compromised vision, or it is the cause of compromised vision, and at times leads to low vision and legal blindness. But I recently met a person whose vision was very sharp and, unusually, was not decreased by the nystagmus. He looked at a small area within the bridge of his nose from a much longer distance than me—more than two feet—and easily stopped his nystagmus by looking there, as the two eyes were in the periphery and the brain was able to notice both. If your vision is good, you can look in a mirror in strong or dim light, from two or three feet, without any problem. If your vision is poor, then look in the mirror from only an inch or less, in only strong light.

The result of looking between the two eyes is productive; however, if you look at one eye, you will not see the flutter because the eye will move with the nystagmus. As you do the aforementioned exercise, you can also move your hips in a rotating motion without moving your head, and this can help to gradually reduce the flutter. Slowing down nystagmus happens with focusing as well, so all the exercises that involve shifting can make a very big difference. The red-and-green-glass exercises can also help to reduce nystagmus. Many people with nystagmus might experience an increase when they are upset or angry or anxious. Palming is helpful, as is sitting or lying in the dark and touching your eyelids ever so gently to feel the flutter with your fingertips; this feeling can slow down the nystagmus. When you touch your eyelids, breathe deeply and count eight slow breaths as you do it. And then palm. When you have finished palming, touch your eyelids again to see if the movement has calmed down. If you follow these recommendations thoroughly, you will greatly decrease your nystagmus in anywhere from a few months to a few years, depending on conditions.

One of the best exercises I did for nystagmus was standing in front of a mirror, where I would put my nose almost on the mirror and move my hips in a rotating motion in both directions. It made a huge difference. I would look between the reflection of my eyes because, if I looked at any one eye, the movement of the eye would not be seen by me. Looking between my eyes helped me see the movement in the periphery and slowed down the nystagmus. I moved my hips in a rotating motion and had a pelvic tilt, to make it like a J shape and then like an S shape, back and forth, mainly forward and then a little bit backward. This has made a very big difference in terms of loosening my whole body and my posture. As more blood circulated to my head, because my body was loosened, my eyes quieted down. We all know that the eyes move quicker in people with nystagmus when they get very upset. Also, light can disturb them. And that's why sunning is such a good exercise. After sunning for a long time, you may temporarily have a bit more nystagmus, but if you do it enough and, of course, if you couple it with palming, you will find that light sensitivity decreases and your nystagmus slows down. Also, I found that long palming sessions—and those can only be done if your whole body is loose and if you don't have a close-angle glaucoma on top of it—can reduce nystagmus over the course of years. If your vision was not compromised, to slow down or erase nystagmus is a good move for your entire central nervous system. If your vision is compromised, as in 95 percent of all nystagmus cases, these exercises are your path to success, along with all the other exercises. Follow the ten steps in chapter 2 and emphasize palming.

Be optimistic. I remember that when I took my dark glasses out, people thought I was on drugs because my eyes would move involuntarily. But there are moments when people tell me that my eyes are so quiet they don't even move.

Chapter 6

Pathological Conditions

Explanations of, and exercises to combat, cataracts, diabetes,
glaucoma, optic neuritis, detached retinas, vitreous detachment,
macular degeneration, and retinitis pigmentosa

Correcting Cataracts

A cataract, put simply, is a cloudy spot on the lens of one's eye. One theory is that cataracts are the result of a crowding of proteins within the lens, which prevents light from passing through. This, in turn, causes an obstruction that eventually makes vision blur or can make a person completely blind. Another theory is that the water pump, which pumps fluid out of the cells, becomes defective and there is swelling, and therefore crowding of the cells in the lens.

There are two main functions of the lens: to transfer light to the retina and to accommodate light properly. You can see why a cloudy spot on the lens would make seeing difficult. Most people experience fuzziness of vision when they reach their mid-sixties to mid-seventies. Upon visits to their eye doctors, they discover that they have cataracts or opacity of the lens.

There are quite a few reasons for cataracts, including poor nutrition and poor metabolism in the body. It is important, therefore, to eat a balanced, healthy diet and to devote time to regular exercise, especially as we get older.

Many other reasons for cataracts are unknown and, in fact, most people don't really care what the cause of their cataract is, because the medical solution seems to work fine for most people, which is simply to remove the lens. Cataracts occur so regularly that we think it is natural, and there is no way to stop it or to save the lens. If the lens has been removed surgically and an intraocular lens is inserted artificially, most people regain the vast majority of their vision. After all, you do not see with your lens—you see with your retina and your brain.

In fact, that tends to be the treatment we like these days. We like to remove parts that are not essential to our daily functions, and either replace them or live without them; then we hail conventional medicine for being able to do it. While I'm happy that cataract surgeries exist, especially because some people cannot manage their cataracts, and the lens needs to be removed anyway, I would like to propose that in 80 percent of cases, when cataracts begin they can be stalled and even stopped for dozens of years, if not eliminated altogether. Moreover, cataracts can be prevented. In modern life the lens does not have the chance to function fully. It becomes thick and opaque because it doesn't move the way it was designed by nature to move.

With the exception of operating on kids, if their lens is opaque in infancy, and where medicine has proven great relief to many children, we need to fight for every lens when cataracts begin. My feeling is that, if we did this, most of the people destined for cataract surgery these days would never actually have it. Often, surgery makes the eyes even worse because it causes scar tissue to build up on the lens capsule. Other times, we have glaucoma attacks that could blind the eye, or there is bleeding in the retina as a result of cataract surgery. There is also the possibility of retinal detachment, especially if somebody has very severe nearsightedness at first, which is called high myopia. It takes only a few weeks to heal the eye but every surgery, to some extent, weakens the body and in this case can weaken the eye, unless you completely heal from it. And that's one of the things that eye exercises may help you do, because, over time, your eye health can get worse as a result of removing your lens, in spite of the miracle that when your lens is removed and an intraocular lens is put in, your vision appears to be extremely clear, as if you gained back years of clarity. Nevertheless, it is at the expense of a vital part of your eye.

One of my patients, Brett, had diabetes. His left eye was operated on successfully and was at 20/20 vision. When his right eye was operated on, he expected to have 20/20 but became blind. I had partial success with Brett's right eye using light therapy, but his doctor negated the results and

Brett lost the small progress he had made with me. Doctors' suggestions can be very powerful. For that reason, I failed in my therapy with Brett, and it was heartbreaking because I liked this wonderful person, and I wanted very much to succeed with him.

On the other hand, one of my best friends and clients, Hannan, had one eye that was sighted and the other nearly blind. We worked for ten years and were able to get the blind eye to see somewhat, and the sighted eye to see better than he had seen since childhood. Then Hannan went to Bascom Palmer, one of the best eye hospitals in the United States, and had cataract surgery. There were complications in the surgery itself. But, after a four-and-a-half-hour surgery, which should have lasted for only forty minutes, his vision became 20/25, which is 95 percent of 20/20, to the amazement of all attending physicians.

We never know what's going to be the result of a medical procedure. Sometimes it's worse than we imagine it would be, like Brett, who had expected to see 20/20 in his right eye. Brett's doctors didn't notice that his calf had to be amputated from the knee down due to diabetes-related gangrene, and that his circulation couldn't possibly be the same when they operated on his right eye. Therefore, his response was not nearly as positive as it was the first time around. But in the case of Hannan, where the physicians were sure there would not be any positive results from the surgery, it was Hannan's insistence that caused them to do the surgery after the cataract was in place for a great many years. He ended up seeing 20/25. What an amazing dichotomy: when they expect to succeed, they fail; when they expect to fail, they succeed.

When one eye overworks and the other eye underworks because of a cataract, the brain works very hard to suppress the information that the underworking eye brings to it. The strain is immeasurable. The eye that overworks becomes fatigued; the eye that underworks becomes weak.

When looking into the distance with cataracts, it's important that you wave your hands quickly to the side and massage around your eye to make it easier. And if the light is hard on you, do sunning for at least five minutes before you look into the distance, and then see if it becomes easier for you. If the light bothers you, put the obstruction glasses over your strong eye, look into the distance with your weaker eye, count twelve different points in the distance, then look at some that are closer, maybe about a quarter of the distance. Next, come visually closer still, another quarter of the distance. Then take the glasses off and again look with both eyes, wave your hands quickly to the side, and massage gently around your eyebrows and cheekbones. Now determine if your sensitivity to light has decreased. When it does, it means that your brain is looking around the obstruction of the cataract and starting to make the lens much more flexible. In that way, you can postpone cataract surgery, and stall the cataract from spreading and expanding.

I'll never forget the patient who came to me with the beginning of a cataract. Nine years later, her doctor said to her, "keep doing what you're doing, your cataract has not changed a bit." That is most likely what will happen to you. If you have the beginning of a cataract, and you are diligent about the ten steps, plus these exercises, it will not change and your vision will remain with a little bit of sensitivity. This should make you feel very satisfied.

So, if your cataract is only beginning to form, this is a good time to work on it. Our statistics are better with cataracts that are just beginning. It may not even mature for many years. You might have an intensive amount of exercises where you can spend up to forty minutes a day on distance viewing.

Sometimes we have to give up on our lens, but often, if we can maintain the lens and not allow it to be opaque, we will affect both our physical and mental sense of being in a positive way. We will feel powerful. We'll break all boundaries of what's possible, because everyone believes you need to have cataract surgery. But with this work, with the intensity of looking into the distance, with palming, with all the ten steps that we have talked about, you will find that you may be able to control your cataracts.

If you experience a cataract, my advice is simply to work on yourself, first with the exercises recommended in this chapter. Remember to refer back to chapter 4 for specific instructions for each exercise. The goal is to get both eyes to work together, and to get the weaker eye to pull its fair share and not get dominated by the stronger eye. Only if your self-care fails to achieve the desired results should you seek help from surgeons.

Exercise Program for Cataracts

Look into the Distance: 30 minutes daily, three intervals of 10 minutes, or 20 minutes once and 10 minutes once.

Look at Details: 10 minutes daily.

Palming: 60 minutes daily.

Bounce and Catch: 10 minutes daily.

A note about cataract surgery: If you are considering cataract surgery, the purpose of doing these exercises is to see whether you can postpone or even cancel the surgery. When you do this program, you should ask yourself if you are improving. If you are, postpone the surgery.

Many people have improved or have stopped the progression of the cataract, so they didn't need the surgery. Some, however, have not improved. If you are one of those who have not improved, and your vision is still poor, a surgery may be indicated. A few weeks after the surgery is done, you can resume eye exercises, and it will benefit your eyes and your vision. I found that some people only want to heal themselves holistically, even if they see extremely poorly and it compromises their life. My recommendation always is a balanced approach. If you cannot heal your vision holistically, then fix it allopathically to help you live fully.

But even for those who did not improve, the fact that they did the exercises was helpful anyway. So don't stop the exercises even if you did not succeed in stopping the cataract. These exercises are good for the overall health of the eye. That is your goal: not to avoid surgery, but rather the health of the eye. If you can prevent surgery, great, and that happens to more than half of the people who follow this program.

We work very hard from infancy to early childhood to create balanced use of the two eyes. Pediatric ophthalmologists understand how important it is to create bilateral vision. What puzzles me, however, is that most ophthalmologists will correct one eye to see near with cataract surgery and one eye to see far. This correction is an error and it goes completely against nature's will for the eyes to work together. It strains the eye and creates tension all over the body.

The best solution to request from your surgeon is for both eyes to be corrected to see well from far away, and with glasses to see well from close-up. With time and exercise, maybe you won't need the glasses.

Note: Remember to work these exercises into the entirety of your day. Don't do an hour and a half all at once. Pace out the exercises so that you are working on your vision all the time, as a matter of habit. Habits determine your destiny.

Extra Exercise for Cataracts: Bounce and Catch

For this exercise you will need the opaque piece of paper to tape to the bridge of your nose, a ball and, if possible, a trampoline. If you are not able to find a trampoline, or if your physical condition prevents you from using one, you can simply try running in place instead of bouncing. The point of bouncing is to distract your mind and body while you practice the exercise, and to engage your peripheral and central vision in a dynamic and different way.

Figure 6.1. The point of bouncing is to distract your mind and body while you practice the exercise.

Simply put the paper on the bridge of your nose so it blocks the central vision of the strong eye, and play catch with someone while you bounce. Wave one hand to the side, above, and also below the eye that is obstructed. Make sure that you can see your hand only peripherally. Bounce and catch for five minutes, then take a break and sun for one minute. Then bounce and catch for another five minutes. Now take the piece of paper off and see how different the world looks. Notice a bigger periphery expanding around you. Notice the intensity of color and shape. It is also helpful to try this exercise with the paper taped to the bridge of your nose from your forehead down to your chin, like in the Melissa Exercise.

Correcting Diabetes

Diabetes is a condition caused when the body cannot produce insulin, or does not utilize insulin in the right way. Insulin is actually a hormone. Insulin's basic function is to transfer glucose, a form of sugar, into the body's cells. There is also a tendency for patients with diabetes to experience poor blood flow.

Poor blood flow can lead to major difficulties in the body, and in extreme cases, heart problems and loss of limbs. Today, we are very aware of how important proper blood flow is to the visual system. Because of poor blood flow to the eyes, some diabetic patients get cataracts, retinopathy, and neovascularization, which are very similar to conditions related to high blood pressure. They lead to continuous bleeding in the retina, which could lead to blindness.

Poor blood flow leads to a response in the retina where new vesicles are formed. This response is very useful in every other part of the body. For example, if you lie down for a month, unable to walk because of a serious illness, and then stand up, at first you'd have pain, partly because you don't have enough blood flow to your legs. Very quickly, the body would form capillaries to bring you circulation, sometimes called "collateral circulation." If your main arteries are clogged or not functional in any way, when the main arteries open up, those vesicles (the capillaries) will degenerate, and the main blood vessels will take over. So, the second or third time that you stand, your legs won't hurt.

Because of diabetes, high blood pressure, or other systemic problems, you do not get enough blood flow to the retina, and the body will form capillaries to nourish the retina. Many times those capillaries are defective; they leak and destroy the sensitive and small photoreceptive cells.

To prevent diabetic attacks, always carry fruits or seeds wherever you go so you can have healthy snacks if there is a rise in your sugar level. More importantly, learn to exercise in a way that brings more blood flow to your whole body and prevents lack of blood flow to your head and retinas.

A twenty-two-year-old woman named Marla, with type 1 diabetes, came to my office. She had already lost a tremendous amount of vision in her left eye due to diabetes and was about to lose a lot in her right eye. She was scheduled for a vitrectomy, a surgical procedure where the vitreous body is removed from the eye in order to protect the retina and to prevent tearing of the retina. While some vitrectomies are very successful in saving eyesight, at times it's the reason for blindness. Therefore, whether or not you know anything about this surgery, you can come to your own conclusion about its success rate. In Marla's case, I thought it best that she not proceed with the surgery and emphatically suggested so.

Because I was so scared of her condition I got her to sign a very long disclaimer—which she was afraid of—since I did not want to take responsibility for the outcome. Regardless, she decided to have the surgery a few days after we met, and it caused her almost absolute blindness in her right eye. Vision in her left eye remained, but a quarter of the left eye simply was not able to see. Consequently, she underwent many laser treatments.

Marla then took my whole training course, which was very helpful to her. I did a lot of *tapotement* massage with her, where I would tap on every bony part of her body, especially her vertebrae. As a result, more and more blood started to be formed because there had been poor blood formation in her bones. We lose red blood cells but we also form red blood cells. The cycle of life and death is within our bodies; it's a beautiful activity. And so Marla started having better coloration.

Unfortunately, even though she did many exercises, she still had terrible vision in her left eye and hardly any in her right eye. So we did an amazing exercise. I gave her a strong flashlight—a pen light—which she held with her right hand and waved very close to her right eye—between her nose and her eye—while reading the eye chart with her left eye. Gradually, she began to read better and better. We did it individually, and we did it in the training course, and her vision improved from 20/400 (5 percent, uncorrectable—where she thought she would have to use special instruments for people who are very visually challenged to see screens) to 20/40. Ultimately, she became a bookkeeper for the small company her husband ran, finished both undergraduate and graduate courses in psychology, and even had the ability to drive. It was amazing to see. After two years of treatment, at the age of twenty-four, Marla told me that it was the first time since the age of seven that she was able to get a clean bill of health from her physician. And against everyone's advice, she eventually brought children into the world.

I have another story with a happy ending. This one is about a seventy-seven-year-old man called Arthur who used to have a massage school. He had lost a lot of his periphery and thought he had very limited central vision because of repeated diabetic attacks. While Marla's diabetes was type 1, Arthur's was type 2, and he was also insulin-dependent. When he tried to read the eye chart, he couldn't. I understood immediately that, because of major loss of his periphery, he did not know where he was looking with his central vision. So I got him to wave his hands to the side quickly, and after doing sunning and palming, he was able to track letters in front of him. Then, noticing his periphery, it was possible for him to find where he was looking. The periphery is that important, because the central periphery can help the central vision to find areas. If you look through a telescope at the stars and you try troubleshooting to find the location of a specific star, you would troubleshoot all night before finding that star; however, if you have another eye open, that eye can help you pinpoint the star you wanted to see. That's exactly what happened with Arthur. By doing peripheral exercises, and just by getting him to wave his hand, we were able to help him use the periphery he was not able to fully use. As a result, he was able to read the chart; in fact, his vision became 20/30, which is 90 percent of 20/20. By stimulating the periphery, he found the letters he wanted to see. With his improved vision, he was able to see details, and his vision kept improving until he had an accident. He was a passenger in a car that had a head-on collision and he went into a coma. When he opened his eyes, he realized his vision was fuzzy and he could not see as well as he used to, so he went back into the coma and died. Arthur had really wanted to see, and for a moment he had a glimpse of light. But when that glimpse disappeared, it seemed he decided his life was not as worthwhile as it should be.

Personally, I believe in the sanctity of life: The more we have it, the better but we can understand that diabetes puts you in a vulnerable state and that you should make a commitment to strengthen yourself. Whether you are twenty-two or seventy-seven, have type 1 or type 2, we should cherish the abilities we have. Be happy with whatever exists for us and move forward. That's my fight for life with many of my patients, and it should be yours as well.

Exercise Program for Diabetes: Up to 2½ Hours Daily (Varies on an Individual Basis)

Massage: at least 20 minutes daily.
Shifting—Looking at Details: at least 10 minutes daily.
Extra Exercise for Diabetes: at least 10 minutes daily.

Many people with diabetes do not develop eye problems. Doing these specific exercises may help the health of the eye. Concentrating on neck and shoulder exercises may prevent eye problems from occurring, because what we need is more blood flow.

The most important thing is to find every way to bring more blood flow to your body because poor blood flow is the secondary problem related to diabetes and is what causes you to lose vision, limbs, and internal organs like kidneys. So the most important thing is blood flow. When you sit and you hold your legs, your knees should be apart and your feet together. The soles of your feet are together and you rub your feet one against the other until they are warm. It is good to do it with socks because they're smoother than bare skin. Over time, you can do it with your bare feet, especially if they don't sweat much. Rub them one against the other while holding your calves, and that warms them up.

Incorporate these exercises into every part of your day. Don't just practice for one hour in the morning, or one hour at night. Find five minutes

Figure 6.2. Bringing more blood flow to the head and retinas.

here and five minutes there, all day, every day. Your diabetes is with you every minute of the day. So you must work constantly to overcome the disadvantages of your diabetes.

For your extra daily exercise, you may choose from any of the following. On some days you might want to practice them all.

Extra Exercises for Diabetes
Tapping

What I found throughout the years is that tapping on all the bones of the body makes a difference with diabetes. After massaging your face, head, eyes, neck, and shoulders, tap rapidly with your fingertips on every bone of your body. You can also stand under the shower and have the shower massager tap on every single bone of your body.

Tapping helps to stimulate blood production.

It's also good to sit down, hold your legs, and rub your feet one against the other. That can help you to create more circulation. The extremities, like feet and hands, are far from the heart. So is the face and, of course, the eyes, and they have a complex vascular system as well. What we want is to bring better blood flow to everywhere in the body. Blood flow is what nurtures the body. The better the blood flow, the more vital, vibrant, and happy we become.

Whenever you massage your body, you have to massage toward the heart. Start by massaging your feet, then your calves, then your thighs in a rotating motion. Then massage your buttocks with your palms; use your fingertips to massage your inguinal area to loosen up the tension in the hips. Then massage your abdominal area firmly, but with some gentleness, and in a rotating motion toward the heart. Massage your chest and tap on the bones in your chest. Next, massage your forehead and then your entire head. This massage therapy can make a very big difference in terms of the blood flow in your body.

Waving

What often happens with diabetes is that you have a major blind spot in your retina. If this is happening to you, hang an eye chart on the wall at eye level, and wave your hand quickly in the area of the blind spot while looking with the healthy areas at the eye chart.

For this exercise, the point is to go back and do all the other eye chart exercises while waving your hand in the area of the blind spot. Review all the exercises in the rest of the book and do them with the stronger eye while you wave your hand quickly in the blind spot.

Patch the Strong Eye

If you have a small damaged portion in one of your retinas, wear a patch on your strong eye and, in front of your weaker eye, place a piece of paper with a small opening in the area of blindness. Then go for a walk around your yard or somewhere else safe. This will force the weakest part of your eye to do all the work.

If you cannot see anything this way, go into a dark room with your strong eye patched, and put blinking lights in front of the weak eye until you begin to experience some sensation of light in the blind spot. Refer to the section on glaucoma below for suggestions on using blinking lights.

Physical Exercises for Diabetes

If your retina did not detach and if you have the body capacity to do so, stand and lift your heels from the ground, while your toes are on the ground, and move your legs as quickly as possible. So you bend and straighten your knees while one foot is up and one foot is down.

Then, quickly lift your toes up while keeping your heels on the ground, dozens of times, and then lift your legs up and stamp on the floor dozens of times. You can start with a soft carpet and then move to a hard floor. The idea is to rattle and shake the bones. This is also a good exercise for osteoporosis, but it's primarily for diabetes. And that is in

Figure 6.3. Lift your heels up, alternating as quickly as possible, then lift your toes. The idea is to rattle and shake the bones.

addition to massage. Also, anyone who has diabetes must walk every day. In the morning, a brisk walk, never less than half an hour, is suggested; in the evening, take a slow walk. This is very important because it gets your blood to flow. Any physician will tell you to do exactly that unless your body cannot handle it.

A Note about Laser Treatments

I would like to discourage you from having too many laser treatments. Many concerned physicians do preventive laser treatments where they basically scar a big portion of the retina to prevent rubeosis, or bleeding in the retina. But if you improve your blood flow, there will be no rubeosis.

Too many laser treatments can weaken the retina and can blind too many parts of it. So while I respect and accept the use of laser treatments to stop continuous bleeding once it occurs, I would like you to aggressively embrace exercises, movement, and dietary change, and to work on damaged areas, in order to help the parts that are not damaged.

These days, doctors use injections to stop bleeding. While injections of Lucentis and other future medications may be effective and less damaging than laser treatments, they still have some damaging effect. My recommendation is to do the injections only when there is bleeding, and not to do it otherwise. Exercise to increase the blood flow, and you will decrease the bleeding.

Cataracts and Diabetes

If you do have cataract surgery, pay attention to your general blood flow, and demand to be checked by the doctor every two hours after the surgery. Doctors hate to be patronized by patients, but don't worry about it. Your health comes first. Make sure that you are being tested every two hours and, if you are, let them test you for bleeding and for any compromise of your retina or optic nerve.

Keratoconus

Keratoconus is a disease that affects the structure of the cornea, the clear tissue covering the front of the eye, which thins and changes to a more conical shape than the more normal gradual curve. The bulge can cause substantial distortion of vision in either eye, and can even affect the patient's ability to drive a car or read normal print when it afflicts both eyes. Estimates of the prevalence for keratoconus range from 1 in 500 to 1 in 2,000 people.

When the cornea becomes irregular, it creates a lot of astigmatism, and with time it changes shape to the extent that we can no longer see well. In the past, doctors used to think that a corneal transplant from a donor was all that was needed to solve the problem. The theory, however, proved unsuccessful because they discovered that rejections of the cornea can be pretty massive and lead to blindness in many cases. Furthermore, using immunosuppressants to suppress the immune system, which would fight a new cornea, can lead to many diseases. Consequently, doctors are a little bit more conservative in replacing corneas these days. Remember, most of the diopters we get come from light breaking on the cornea. The cornea itself does not have as much aptitude as the lens (it is not as powerful as the lens of the eye) but has more diopters within the eye because light breaks first in the cornea. We'd do better to use the old treatment of medicine from the 1980s: hard contact lenses. In the meantime, we need a lot of self-massage around the eyes every day. Start by first massaging from the bridge of your nose to your temples (over your eyebrows), then from your nose to your ears (over you cheekbones). Next, find the grooves in your cheekbones and eyebrows; massage them and they will loosen up. Wear the hard contact lenses only three to four hours a day, leaving a day or two off per week, in order to rest the eyes; otherwise, they will eventually prove bad for the eyes. If you follow these procedures, you may postpone or prevent corneal replacement for many years.

Today, what bothers me more than anything else is that some people get keratoconus due to unsuccessful LASIK surgery, which I oppose because it damages the eyes so much that, even with glasses, their vision is beyond repair. All ten steps of the eye exercises are good for keratoconus, but the emphasis should be on massage. In fact, I had the pleasure of working with several people who were able to prevent corneal transplants as a result of several months of massage in dark rooms.

Charles was a man in his forties who came to me with keratoconus in the 1980s, and he tried to use a contact lens that would change the shape of his eye. But the contact lens caused him a tremendous amount of pain, so both his optometrist and ophthalmologist strongly recommended a corneal replacement. He came to me because his wife was a student in one of my training courses and was very impressed with my work on her back. So I massaged him and we practiced all ten steps of the eye exercises, especially the reading and shifting work that we do in this book. The massage around his eyes relaxed him enough that his contact lenses fit him just fine. In fact, his cornea even changed shape. Eight months later, both his optometrist and ophthalmologist told him that surgery would not be necessary. He still had keratoconus but to a much lesser extent, making surgery a drastic, unnecessary step.

Interestingly, when Charles asked if he could share with them how he had improved his eyes, neither of them cared to hear about it. It is the fate of my work that this keeps recurring. When people improve to an extent that science would have been interested to discover, even doctors who recognize that improvement have a hard time admitting that something other than what most people who serve medical science think could make a difference. Medicine cannot prevent keratoconus from advancing. All doctors can do is change the cornea and fit you with very strong glasses to deal with the situation. So I feel so good about Charles because he's doing well till this very day. I wish that more people would join him and get massaged around the eyes, in the dark, and do all ten steps with diligence. Eventually, you will end up improving your vision.

Correcting Glaucoma

Glaucoma is a disease of the optic nerve, often caused by irregular pressure in the eyes, which results in loss of the visual field and, eventually, blindness. Glaucoma can be a scary disease for many people because of this, and also since its symptoms may not be obvious until the disease is quite advanced.

The loss of vision that occurs with glaucoma has a few factors. One is pressure, and another is weakness of the optic nerve and disk. So if you have a very strong optic nerve and disk, even high pressure will not necessarily lead to a loss of vision. But if you have a weak optic nerve and disk, even low pressure could lead to a loss of vision.

For this reason, everyone must be evaluated to determine whether they have a weak or a strong optic nerve and optic disk, before the effects of pressure can be understood and predicted accurately.

The complication here comes from LASIK surgery because it alters the thickness of the cornea, which will alter the perception of pressure, thus making it harder to measure. To date, after LASIK surgery, it is hard to determine what the pressure truly is.

We would like to assume that normal pressure in the eye is above 10 millimeters of mercury (mmHg) and below 20. Anything less than 10 could be too little pressure on the eye. We need pressure in the eye just like a tire needs pressure to maintain its integrity. But, when the pressure mounts, it can destroy weak areas in our eyes. The main area that it destroys is the optic disk, which is rather weak in all of us, but with people who have glaucoma, the weakness of their disk is more pronounced. Reducing pressure would take away the risk of blindness or, at least, of partial blindness.

Statistically, it is true to say that those who have pressure above 30 will most likely lose more vision, but only statistically. In any particular case, it could be that even a pressure higher than 30 does not lead to vision loss. You could also say that some people at a pressure of only 24 or 25 may lose a lot of vision.

The other problem that could easily occur is low-tension glaucoma. With low-tension glaucoma, even having pressure under that which is considered to be desirable for most of us, the optic disk degenerates and is destroyed. The optic disk is the area where the optic nerve connects to the eye; this is a weak and a vulnerable area. When that area has pressure it cannot withstand, the optic disk can be compromised. In some people with completely normal pressure (the 16 mmHg that most of us want to have), the optic disk is still destroyed. This is the prevailing viewpoint. While I agree with it to a point, I believe that it is only a part of what happens. Therefore, the treatment is sometimes ineffective, and can even be dangerous because it only works on the eye pressure without considering other factors.

A few years ago I had the pleasure of working with a bright woman named Lucia, who came all the way from Brazil to San Francisco for two weeks of intensive sessions with me. She came to me with much fear because she had lost 95 percent of her nerve functionality due to glaucoma. The surprising thing about her case was that, after doing the eye exercises and before she even met with me, she gained back the peripheral vision she had lost; her field of vision was almost completely normal—with only one small spot of vision loss—and her acuity was 20/20. I am not the only one who is surprised with such magnificent vision after such significant loss of nerve tissue.

Lucia also told me that several of her family members were afflicted with cardiovascular disease. Knowing that she had this family history, my conclusion from her case was that doing the exercises had increased her blood flow to the remaining nerve tissue, and had improved the situation tremendously. Doctors had offered her a very risky surgery to reduce the pressure, but it would have also posed a big risk to her vision, and she could have lost it completely. Eventually Lucia did the surgery and found it to be useful. So she combined it with doing eye exercises, and it worked well for her.

My ideas of what can help people with glaucoma are:

1. Reduction of pressure (in this I agree with doctors).
2. A balanced use of the two eyes and within each eye.
3. Having sufficient circulation that nourishes the optic nerve.

In Lucia's case, the bodywork we did was just as important as the vision work, and the part of the nerve that is working assumed the work of the nerves that had been destroyed.

The frustrating part of it all is that even when you reduce the pressure to 10 or 11, as many doctors want you to reduce it to, the optic disk may be preserved in some cases, but with others it may continue to erode to the point of destruction, causing damage to the optic nerve. And the feeling shared by medical doctors is that the optic nerve can never regenerate.

In order to reduce pressure in glaucoma, we discovered that if you use one hand to touch an eye that does not have pressure, and the other hand to touch an eye that has pressure, it will decrease the level of pressure in the eye with high pressure. Let me be clear that you don't simply touch your own eyes; either you touch someone else's eye that is soft while your eye is hard, or the other person with a soft eye without high pressure touches his or her eye and your eye. For example, if a family member has high pressure, you first put the fingertips of one of your hands on the closed lid of their afflicted eyeball and the fingertips of your other hand on the lid of the unafflicted eye of another person in your family so you can feel the difference. Then put those same fingertips on your eye. You may be able sense the pressure, because often there is hardness and firmness when there is pressure. Then once again, put your fingertips on the family member's afflicted eye, breathe one hundred deep breaths as you do so, and then touch your eye again and see if, compared with your eye, the afflicted eye you're touching becomes softer. Your best gauge to feel their eye pressure is by feeling the pressure of your own eye. This is a subtle ability. If you reach that ability, you may find that you are able to considerably reduce the pressure of their afflicted eye.

If a family member or a friend went to the ophthalmologist, and they're just about to get pressure-reducing drops but you want to postpone it for a couple of weeks, spend as much as twenty-five minutes to half an hour every day touching both eyes: Touch their afflicted eye and your own unafflicted eye for twelve and a half minutes to fifteen minutes each time. And always remember that the touch has to be very, very gentle. Then determine if the hardness gradually goes down. In a short period of time, the pressure should start to be even between the one who touches and the one who is being touched. The process allows the person being touched to slowly learn, within the mechanism of their own body, how to reduce the pressure in their eyes. It might surprise you that the slightly risen pressure of the eye in the unafflicted person will go back to normal because there's no anatomical reason for that pressure to remain high. This will happen within a very short period of time. On the other hand, the person whose has high pressure may have it return to being high, but it might not be quite as high and may even go down through enough repetition and work with the rest of the exercises for glaucoma.

You need to understand that cell communication can be transferred through your fingers. You're actually educating the eye cells how to change through touch, and they will start to feel how to accomplish better drainage of inner ocular fluid (aqueous fluid) so that the eye can remain soft. Though this concept might seem bizarre, more and more scientists are finding that cell communication *does* exist. And this method is a good way to create cell communication between hands and eyes.

Another way to reduce pressure is through physical exercises like the ones in this chapter, specifically the exercises for neck release. It is significant that sports and low-impact aerobics can often reduce eye pressure. Even when the pressure of low-tension glaucoma is down to 11 or 12, which is desirable among most doctors, those patients may still lose their vision. In summary, balance the use of the eyes and balance the use within each eye, also touching the eye for person-to-person cell communication, and exercises for neck release.

Unlike cataract surgery, about which physicians are very optimistic, physicians continuously see that they cannot fully control glaucoma: not with drops, not with surgery. There is no way to clarify to anyone that reduction of pressure equals reduction of destruction of the optic nerve. And it is clear that most people like to have a simple technical solution to complex problems. Since there seems to be no magic bullet for glaucoma, people live in fear. And that fear is one of the main destructive dangers to our eyes.

The eyes feel this fear. The tissues feel the fear as well, then become much worse. With some of my patients who had temporary improvement in therapy, I sometimes felt that this cloud of fear caused them to deteriorate anyway. With other patients, where the situation seemed to be grave compared to everyone else, their trust in the therapy dramatically improved their vision through the correct exercises and the right knowledge. Positive affirmation can be very useful. You can close your eyes and visualize that the strength of your eyes outpowers any phenomenon that can destroy them. Positive affirmation is 50 percent of your healing process.

When it comes to high pressure in the eyes, all factors must be considered: lack of balanced use of the eyes; stiffness of the neck (which is a result of stiffness of the body); a sense of emotional loss—not just stress, but loss.

A good example is the desire for peace and harmony in a relationship, but never finding it because of resolutions that never come. Similarly, kids of divorced parents feel this when they want to see their parents getting along but never see that happen. There are many different situations that can cause glaucoma, so apply this book in a way that works for your specific situation.

Some people had lost a lot of vision before the practice of these exercises and will do anything they can to keep the vision they already have, and to sharpen it to a great extent. Other people have hardly lost any vision and, therefore, do the eye exercises to prevent any potential vision loss and to sharpen their vision. Some people have only a mild vision loss. Pay attention to the area where your vision is mildly lost, and use the area that is fuzzy or almost blind; this will help you to defend the rest of your visual system. So, apply the book individually to your needs. Take time and pay attention to yourself in a way that works for you.

I will never forget one of my dearest patients, Murray, who had glaucoma. He did well in his therapy with me for a period of seven years. But he took a turn for the worse when his wife died. Issues between him and his wife were never resolved, and that's one of the worst things that happens when a person you love perishes. If a person who was very dear to you did not get along with you, and the problem you had with that person was never resolved, with their death comes a sense of loss without closure. Part of this loss is not processing your inner feelings around the unresolved issues you had with the deceased. Murray had a problem with his wife's senility and the Alzheimer's disease she had developed toward the end of her life. He discovered much anger that she had against some people that she had never brought out during their marital life. It revealed much of her anguish that he had never noticed during her youth. He was struck by the amount of anger and frustration that came out of her when she forgot the present and only remembered the past. And here was a woman who was a world educator and a writer.

When she died, his glaucoma became much worse because his emotional state lacked the stability that he had during most of the marriage. He was also exhausted from trying to keep his wife in as good a shape as he could during the last years of her life. Often, when there is a sense of loss and death, it can lead to loss of vision. A sense of loss or death could result from the absence of anything that you really loved and adored, like relationships, stability, or a home you had liked but from which you had to move. Anything that deep inside leads to an emotional connection and, when it leaves your life without a positive resolution, it could lead to tremendous subconscious tension. That tension reveals itself as a great muscular contraction in your neck. And that neck contraction hampers and disturbs the blood flow to your brain and to your eyes. When it disturbs the blood flow to your brain, you're running a risk of strokes and hemorrhages of the brain cells. When it disturbs the blood flow to your eyes, you run the risk of losing retinal areas and vision, and you run a greater risk of having high pressure in your eyes. Sometimes you have good blood flow to the head, but in the head the blood vessels could be a bit narrow, and the skull could be tight. So letting go of skull tension is very, very important for sufficient blood flow to the optic nerve.

Pearl, who came to me fifteen years ago with good vision in her right eye and challenged vision in her left, was able to preserve her eyesight with my help. But when she started having surgeries, there were side effects, like cataracts that had to be removed, and a retina that became detached after the cataract was removed. Then layers of scar tissue had to be removed after the retinal reattachment surgery, which resulted in the loss of much of the vision in her left eye, but the vision in her right eye was preserved and is still 20/30.

We like to say that working with glaucoma is a work in progress. There are many genes that lead to losses related to glaucoma. These are genes that make the optic nerve weak. So even under normal pressure, you can lose vision. Also, emotions can make your optic nerve weak and your circulation poor. When the circulation to the optic nerve is poor, it could cause you to lose vision as well.

Some people have simple problems with the optic nerve. The blood vessels that bring blood to it become thin, maybe sluggish, and they don't allow for good blood flow, thus leading to destruction of the optic nerve. I've had three patients with destruction of the optic nerve without it being glaucoma, and I was only able to help the third one, who was diligent in doing my exercises. He was able to preserve his vision and even became able to drive.

So it's important for us to know that, while sometimes loss is irreversible, it's usually an issue of blood flow. It calls for opening vessels in the body for better blood flow as well as opening the small vesicles near the optic nerve, which would allow the blood to flow and to nourish it. Good circulation in the body and loosening of the neck to allow good circulation to and within the head makes a very big difference in keeping the optic nerve alive. At the same time, we need to have good use of the retinas.

In the early 1980s I was introduced to a young man, about sixteen years of age, who had a defective heart. His heart was racing at a speed of 104 beats per minute, so he came to my office. I was young then, and my heart—just like in all the textbooks of the time—was 72 beats per minute. With one hand, I touched his heart, and with the other hand, I touched my heart. My assistant, Ellen, was a good nurse with very sharp eyes; I described her previously in the palming section in chapter 2. She measured our pulses within five minutes of my feeling his heartbeat above the seventh rib, and both had become 84 beats per minute. When I took my hands off our chests, our heartbeats changed again. Mine returned to 72, but his only climbed to 94. That was one of the first times I actually experienced how my touch could affect somebody else's bodily function, even though I had believed in it before.

A similar thing happened to me with an infant of two and a half years of age, who had an eye pressure of 27 mmHg, one blind eye due to total retinal detachment after cataract surgery, and one legally blind eye with a pressure of 27. I did many exercises with her, but the pressure remained the same. When I touched her eye and mine, her pressure was reduced to 11. Therefore, touch is amazing in its capacity to help you reduce pressure. It's not a panacea, and you cannot count on it, but it's worth doing. It's important to know that the true panacea is increased blood flow and activity of the eyes.

In many cases, we lose vision to glaucoma. I say "we" because I really identify with my clients and patients. The way we lose more and more is if we don't properly use the vision we have, and quite often we succumb to having less vision without best using what we have. For example, if you see well from both the left and right sides of your eye, but you lost a lot of vision in the center, you may not be using the places that you have. I've seen a woman guided by her husband in spite of having moderately good vision in the two sides of her eyes, and so I taught her to simply move her head gently from side to side in order to see her environment. It often happens that we lose part of our visual field and become so discouraged that we don't use the rest. Then, the part we are left with degenerates from lack of use. If we are encouraged to use what we have, and we use these exercises, we stand a very good chance of gaining back some of the parts of our visual field that still exist. Consequently, your life becomes much better, and you will feel much more in control of it.

When we talk about fear, when people have fear of loss of vision, it leads to paralysis and lesser use of the remaining vision after some loss has occurred. That is, by the way, also true about the rest of the body. In the case of a woman who had multiple sclerosis and was walking with a cane, I found that only one of her toes was really paralyzed and that the rest of her leg was merely stiff. When the stiffness was loosened, she was able to walk much better. And so, discouragement comes to both clients and medical professionals, when some previously functioning body parts have been lost, that that the rest cannot be used either, which eventually leads to further loss. One thing I can say is that more and more therapists in the visual education field are trying to help people engage with the parts of their eyes that still exist and that could work better.

While glaucoma is an organic illness that leads to destruction, to a great extent we have a situation that reflects lack of peace within one's life. I just recently had a client who came from far away to San Francisco, and she went through many difficulties in her life, some of them physical. She had fallen and broken her ankle, and suffered from what's called low-tension glaucoma. So we mainly worked on balanced use of the eyes, along with a request for her to walk long distances. We did all the exercises with the red and green glasses and with the beads and long-distance walk. She brought with her a machine similar to the one used by physicians to measure pressure, and learned that those are the best exercises for her. It's always nice to find out what works best for you. While her work at this point is still in progress, after working with her for a few weeks, her pressure dropped from 19 to 13. Although the pressure of 19 mmHg is excellent for most people, in her case it was a surgery-saver. Her physician wanted to put a structure in her eye that would drain the fluid, but when he saw that her pressure had dropped and her vision was stable, he decided to cancel the surgery. Anytime surgery is avoidable by working on our eyes, we extend visual life. Because surgery is never the final point, you should still pursue this work. Bringing more blood flow to the optic nerve brings more life to the eyes, and that becomes most important.

Special instructions for palming with glaucoma: You should only palm for up to ten minutes at a time. Then wait at least five minutes in between ten-minute sessions. You can do this many times a day. But if you palm too long all in one session, you can experience an increase in pressure. If, for example, you have closed-angle glaucoma and you palm for half an hour all at once, you can have an increase in pressure of 4 mmHg.

Exercise Program for Glaucoma

Peripheral Exercise: 20 minutes daily.

Palming: 6 minutes at a time, three times daily, with at least 5 minutes between sessions.

Sunning: 20 minutes daily.

Headlines (from the section on astigmatism in chapter 4): 10 minutes.

Block the Strong Eye (Tape the medium-size piece of paper onto the bridge of your nose so that it blocks the central vision of your strong eye. Now read with your weaker eye while waving your hand in the periphery of your stronger eye): 10 minutes.

Physical Exercises for Glaucoma: 20 minutes daily.

Note: While working on your eyes, also address your emotional state and create a good emotional environment for yourself. And remember to work on your eyes throughout the day. Always find time here and there to work on healing your vision.

Physical Exercise for Glaucoma

Good thoughts and good prayer can be healing. Visualize that blood is circulating to your retina, making it soft and nurturing to your optic disk. Also visualize that the fluid in its clear form is flowing in the area between the cornea and the macula. Visualize that good blood circulation is nourishing your optic disk and retina. Visualize the blood coming from the back, and from your neck to the back of the head, and nourishing your optic disk. Visualize that blood is flowing into your eye and draining from it. Then visualize that plasma, the white and clear area of the blood, is flowing into the front area of your eye from the cornea to the lens, nourishing both, and draining into the area of your nose. It's amazing how powerful the body is and how much it does all at once. It's not power that belongs to you but to nature, and you are a wonderful guest of nature's within your own body. There is a connection between that power and of all universal powers around you; this connection gives that power a tremendous amount of strength.

The same power that brings rain from the sky and wind to the earth, the same power that is mysterious to all of us and runs the whole universe, is the same power that moves your blood and your fluids. It does so constantly. The more you acknowledge its power and its strength, the better it will work for you. There is a connection between your mind and your soul, and the natural functions of your body. When you have glaucoma, physical exercises are important to prevent the pressure from mounting and growing in your eyes and, in fact, reduce it.

Other exercises are important to preserve your vision. All of them will be pleasant to do and a pleasure to work with. When you work on your body, you work for the purpose of having fun with it, and it is a pleasure to do the work. When you have that feeling, it's going to be wonderful to heal your glaucoma and to overcome it. It will create a better connection between you and your internal forces, and it will help you to tune in to the forces of the universe. It's probably the best antidepressant you can ever have.

Exercises for Glaucoma

Sunning is one of the best eye exercises you can do for glaucoma, because it temporarily reduces your eye pressure. It also contracts the pupils and creates better fluid flow within your eyes. So, for the time that you do it, your pressure is being reduced. And the reduction of pressure will last if you can also release the tension in your neck. This exercise will help you do that.

If you are a typical glaucoma patient, if such a thing exists, most likely you have a very tight neck. Tension of the neck, to a great extent, is a result of mental stress as well as physical stress, but not in all cases. Nevertheless, I have found that many people who have a tendency for glaucoma exacerbate that tendency with either injury or tension in the neck.

It's important for you to know that you need to work on your neck, first spiritually, then mentally. It's good to write about your thoughts and feelings in a journal. Then meet with a good friend or maybe with a psychotherapist who can help you. Hopefully, with holistic inclinations, you will see your whole life and all phenomena as one unified experience.

Sometimes, it's important for you to take a good vacation or to do things that can improve your life. For example, let yourself be drawn into having a relationship if you don't have one, or into finding a way to get out of your shell of loneliness if you are lonely. And, if you have a relationship, allow yourself to examine it and to find out if you really spend enough time with your partner; allow yourself to develop good communication skills with your partner in order to bring smoothness into your life. It's important to do the work that will help you to feel that you are doing well emotionally and that you're advancing yourself spiritually. Then, you just may find yourself in a whole new place of physical self-improvement with these exercises. Often, the exercises will bring back emotional phenomena, which you'll want to deal with whenever they come, in order to reach a place of neutrality and tranquility.

These days, many people do not understand the value of neutrality. Somebody jokingly wrote me a postcard that said, "Meir, never tell me to relax. My tension is the only thing that holds me together." That's why many people function with tremendous amounts of tension and think it's good: because they always do it. Life is much happier with less tension. In a place of relaxation, you feel security and love in the universe.

Now, while facing the sun with your eyes closed, continue to move your head from side to side and stroke your cheekbones, massaging around your eyes and nose. Massaging the areas around your eyes is very helpful for relaxation. Quite often, the tension of the eyes leads to squinting, as I've mentioned in the beginning of this book. That is a tension that you want to undo. When you take away squinting, you take away pressure, and when you take away pressure, the eye becomes healthy.

Move your head from side to side. Then move your head up and down while moving from side to side. Your chin points upward toward the sky and downward toward your chest. You should move your head up and down four times, from the edge of your shoulder to the middle, and four times from the middle of your shoulder to the edge. This really helps to loosen up your neck and to create more space between the first vertebra and the crown. After doing this forty times, palm for thirty seconds. Then you should do it another forty times, if you can relax while performing the exercise. (No longer massage around the eyes, because it's not safe to do this when you move the head up and down.) Just move your head up and down as you're facing the sun with your eyes closed. Then you palm again. Do this exercise a third time and then palm yet again for thirty seconds to a minute. Next, move your head from side to side and massage your eyebrows and cheekbones. Now, go into the shade or sit in a dark room and palm for six to eight minutes at a time, with an emphasis on slow, deep breathing.

You can also take the glow-in-the-dark ball into a very dark room. It normally energizes with light, so you can bring the ball into the sun during sunning to make it glow. In our school we use a closet or the accessible restroom and close the door to make it very, very dark. Then, as a group, we throw the ball from person to person. At first the room seems to be awfully dark, but with time even the pale light of the glowing ball in the dark gets us to see the room much better. Then you go out and do sunning again. That leads to tremendous movement within your eyes because when you do sunning, your pupils constrict. When you throw the ball in the dark, your pupils relax. So when you do sunning and then the throw ball in the dark about six or seven times, each time for two or three minutes, you will find that all of a sudden, your pupils respond better to the light and constrict better in the light. Consequently, the light bothers you less and you respond better to the dark because your pupils expand quicker and better in a dark room. For this reason, you see better in a dark room; it becomes much lighter and clearer.

Now bend your knees and straighten them again. Try to bring your knees to the level of your abdomen or chest (this depends on how flexible your hips are), while moving your head from side to side. If balance is an issue, hold onto a wall or a chair as you do this exercise. Make sure that you don't fall while doing it.

Now march in place and move your head from side to side while moving your legs up and down, in order to pump more blood into the head and loosen the neck. If you have good balance, as you move your legs up and down and move your head from side to side, massage your hands. Especially massage the place in the palm that is between the thumb and the index finger. If it's hard for you to do three things at once (gently and steadily moving your head from side to side all the way, moving your legs up and down, and massaging your palm), you can do two things. Massage your hand and move your head from side to side, or move your head from side to side and just move your legs up and down. These are things that can help bring more blood flow and calm your nervous system; don't strain to do them.

After massaging your palm, and while moving your legs up and down, just simply move your head from side to side twenty or thirty times; then go indoors and palm for eight minutes. When you relax from the palming, you will have time to loosen up your neck.

Before doing neck exercises, determine how well your neck moves from side to side. Lie down on your back, bend your knees, and move your head from side to side about ten times to sense the neck's restriction. Then, once you have an idea of the range of motion available to you, begin these exercises so that, at first, you stay within your comfortable range of motion. Gradually, this range of motion should increase over time. Also, with all these neck exercises, you should strive for fifteen to twenty repetitions on each side for each exercise.

Figure 6.4. Bend your knees, stretch out your arms, and turn to face your left hand (a). Reach your right arm across to and past the left hand (b).

Now lie on your back, bend your knees, stretch your arms, and look at one hand; let's say the right hand. Take the left hand and bring it all the way to the right and, in fact, pass it. Stay there for one deep breath. Keep your head looking at the right while bringing the left hand all the way to the left. The shoulder will then stretch in two ways. For one, it will stretch in the back muscles, the trapezius and the rhomboids, in order to bring the arm forward. The second time, when you bring your arm back to where it was, the pectoral muscles of the chest will stretch, and chest muscles as well as back muscles are directly connected to neck muscles.

Then move your head to the opposite side and do exactly the same exercise with your right hand reaching to the left. You can let your legs move after your arm if that's what your body needs to do to complete the stretch. Repeat the exercise thirty-five times. Then move your head from side to side; 90 percent of the people who do this feel that the neck is looser when they do it. Then put your hands behind your head and lift up your head without the neck helping you. Do it six or seven times. See if you can let go of your neck and just let your hands do the work. Then put one hand on your forehead and move your head from side to side, with your hand on your forehead and your neck loosening.

Another great exercise for the neck is to walk backward. Do it for four hundred or five hundred yards a day, every day. Look over your shoulder from time to time, which is also a great exercise to stretch your neck. At the same time, it's good for you to work with a friend, at least once a week, although a few times a week is even better. Your friend will put his or her legs on your shoulders and stretch your neck.

Another wonderful exercise for the neck is to sit on a chair, put your chin on your chest, and then slowly bend down until you touch the floor. Then straighten up with your legs first, and then with your whole back. Now do the same thing from a standing position. Bend over, putting your chin on your chest, and slowly bend down, vertebra by vertebra. Put your hand on the floor and, only after you do, sit on the chair while still bending. Then, keeping your chin on your chest and your hands on the floor, you straighten.

Figure 6.5. Sit cross-legged and move your whole body in a rotating motion (a). Let your head roll loosely as your body rotates (b). Make big, full circles with your body (c).

Next, if you do not have a tendency for retinal detachment, which many people with glaucoma do not, you can also sit cross-legged and move your whole body in a rotating motion. Sit on the floor with your legs crossed. Put your hands on your knees. Bend forward and rotate your whole body in a broad circular motion, bending at the waist, rotating all the way around one way and then the other, feeling your spine elongate and your neck stretch. Go both directions: left, then right. Now put both hands on your right leg and lean forward so that your forehead touches your right knee. Lean forward, then straighten back up. Do this five times. Then put both hands on your left knee. Bend forward so your forehead touches your left knee, then straighten back up. Do this five times. Now bend at the waist and rotate your whole body again.

Figure 6.6. Rotate your head to the left and to the right several times and then in a circular motion on the floor.

Next (as long as you don't have retinal detachment), get down on all fours and put your forehead on the floor. Rotate your head to the left and to the right, keeping your forehead in contact with the floor. Go right and left slowly, gently breathing in and out. Now, keeping the crown of your head in contact with the floor, rotate your head in a circular motion on the floor. You might just feel your scalp coming to life. Move the crown of your head on the floor, in a rotating motion, breathing deeply and slowly. If this hurts, simply modify the pressure on your head by using your hands to support your weight. Go back to sitting cross-legged again, and move your body once more in a rotating motion, bending at the waist. Take your time and breathe. Really feel how relaxed your neck is becoming.

Next, you will want to sit down on the floor with your back against a wall, and your knees bent in front of you. If for any reason (if you have a very large belly) you have a hard time bending your knees, sit cross-legged instead. Otherwise, bend your knees. If you want, you can put a small pillow behind the middle of your back, underneath your shoulders, to make it more comfortable.

First, move your head all the way to the left so that you are stretching your neck muscles as you breathe deeply. Tap your fingers on the stretched muscles on the opposite side of your neck. Massage the neck muscles with your thumb and fingers. Now turn your head in the other direction, stretching the other side of your neck, and do the same thing on the opposite side, tapping the stretched muscles with your fingers, and then massaging that side of the neck with your thumb and fingers.

Figure 6.7. Tap your fingers on the stretched muscles on the opposite side of your neck.

After several repetitions on both sides, interlace your fingers underneath your knees and bend forward until your forehead touches your knees, and straighten back to the wall about twenty times. This loosens up the middle of your back.

Put your hands on your knees and push your legs to one side and then the other, using only the strength of your hands, not your legs. Push your knees to the left and then to the right. You will feel yourself starting to scoot forward and to slip down on the wall; that's okay. Just pause and scoot yourself back up into the seated position with which you started. Start over again from the beginning, turning your head from side to side. You may find that your neck is much looser now.

It's also a very good idea to close your eyes and to put a warm towel over them. Moisten the towel with warm water or with herbal tea; there is one in particular called eyebright tea, which has been very effective for me. For those of you who use computers, look into the distance and apply warm and cold towels to your eyes after using the computer. If there is not enough time for both types of towels, apply only cold towels to take away the inflammation. Apply warm and cold towels over your eyes at least once a week.

Figure 6.8. Turn your head from side to side.   Figure 6.9. Push your knees to the left and then to the right.

Another thing that my clients like very much is the steam machine that my sister, who owns health spas, has donated to our school. Steam in a dark room can be very relaxing when you have your eyes closed. While not a necessity, this is a nice luxury, and people who have experienced the steam machine, along with cold towels around their eyes, say they felt wonderful. It's one of the reasons that so many people love to have facials, which are very useful for relaxation.

Reduction of pressure, moisture in the eyes, clear vision, a loose neck, and a sense of well-being are all good indicators of improvement. You should create a peripheral chart like the sample in this book, with a point in the middle and many numbers at the side of that chart. Copy it somewhat larger, and each time see how the chart looks. If you found that, let's say, the right part of the chart is not clear but it became clearer after you did exercises, you know that your periphery is better. You can have some stress when you're being measured at a doctor's office. I have heard of

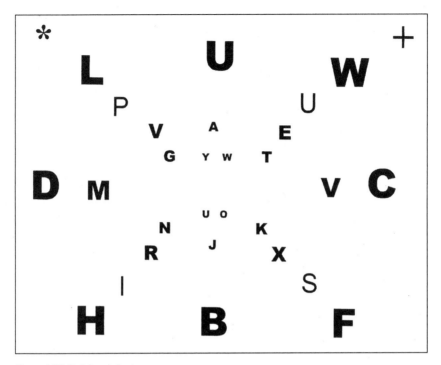

Figure 6.10. Peripheral chart.

people who were measured by one machine that showed their periphery was diminished, then being measured by another machine that showed their periphery was doing well. Sometimes, the machine is accurate and we should listen to what we're being told; however, it's usually best to measure yourself at home, to determine if you see better. In summary, work on your periphery, work on areas that were lost, and work on central areas as well. Balanced use within each eye is very important, and so is doing the Melissinia Exercise.

Please look back at the Melissa and Melissinia exercises in chapter 5, and also look ahead at the Melissinia exercise in "Correcting Optic Nerve Damage" section.

These exercises are essential for reduction of tension. After doing these exercises every day for a period of around three months, measure your pressure and see if it went down. If so, you may be able to prevent the need to use eyedrops, as long as your ophthalmologist does not oppose the idea; at least, you may be able to reduce them gradually with supervision. Find a friendly ophthalmologist or optometrist who is willing to measure your pressure frequently, ideally twice a week, so you will know that you are on the right path.

Neurological Problems and Vision

In my forty-four years of work—and I've been doing this work before I was even seventeen—I've encountered many unusual phenomena. Some are diagnosed, some are not. For instance, I met a lovely Austrian woman with an unusual nerve disease for which a diagnosis has only recently been found, but it's still not in the books. She was affected all over her body: she suffered from dizziness, repeated headaches, a general weakness of the body, and a strange phenomenon where her right eye saw the world in a reduced way; it would see things smaller than they really are, while her left eye saw the actual size. And she would see them smaller through the side of her left eye. Bodywork, sunning, and palming helped, but what helped her the most was the work with red and green glasses. The card games with the red and green glasses, the light work with the card games, and the Melissinia Exercise all made a difference. What surprised me was that as we did the Melissinia—patching the right eye and putting three different sizes of paper over the left eye—sometimes she would find it relieving, but other times she would find that it caused her headaches. So we worked in two different ways. We used a thin piece of paper, threw the ball above her head, and got her to catch it. Then we did the same with the medium-size paper, and also with the large-size paper, which is about three-eighths of an inch wide. Next, we took the same three pieces of paper, and first patched her right eye with the small piece of paper and waved the blinking light (called a magic wand) in the dark. This was repeated with the medium and large pieces of paper. Gradually, we reduced the size of those papers.

We discovered later on that her headaches were reduced when we also patched her left eye, which was the weaker one, and worked a little on the stronger eye with the same exercises. First came the ball that we threw in the sun or bright daylight. Then came the thin paper, which was one-eighth of an inch; the wider, which was two-eighths of an inch;

and the widest, three-eighths of an inch. We learned that when we put the longest piece of paper—and also the widest one—in front of her left eye and then in front of her right eye, and used the three thin pieces of paper, her headaches disappeared. We also learned that when we used the large piece of paper, which we call a "Melissa" and which did not block the whole eye like a patch would, and put Melissinias on the other eye, it worked better for her. It surprised us because we were trying to get only one eye to work at a time, where only different parts of that eye would work. But we found that even when the other eye would work a little bit, it made it possible for her brain to have a sense of expansion. In essence, we were affecting different parts of the brain—the thalamus and the occipital lobe—through working on the eye. By blocking different areas of one eye, but as long as there is some openness in the other eye, there is activity in different peripheral areas of the eye. Therefore, balanced use of the eye is very important, especially for a very unusual neurological condition.

Meanwhile, her situation has improved amazingly because she works on herself several hours a day. Her exercises include crawling, which balances the use of different parts of the brain, and falling from side to side, which loosens up the neck and uses parts of the brain that are not normally used.

The exercise for the eyes that we call the Melissinia is something everyone who reads this book should do. In fact, my recommendation is that, when you read this book, don't look only for what would help your case; instead, look at everyone else's cases and see which exercises might be relevant to your particular situation. I don't know of one person who has not sharpened their vision simply by practicing the Melissinia, because more parts of the visual system are working. So, while patching one eye and throwing the ball from area to area is a very important thing, using a small piece of paper and then larger ones is just as significant.

As in the section on glaucoma, working with a glowing ball in the dark, in combination with sunning, was very powerful for a woman named Magdalena. It was very helpful because it affects the pupils, and the pupils affect the nervous system. The autonomic nervous system comprises two opposing systems: one is more active and includes the fight-or-flight mechanism (sympathetic); the other is more relaxing and includes the digestive mechanism (parasympathetic). The latter is compromised through long-term stress—emotions that don't resolve themselves in any way—and through our lifestyle, like looking at computers a lot and being in unfavorable light conditions. The activity of the pupils relaxes and balances that system. And, for that reason, the body can function much better with the autonomic nervous system.

Correcting Optic Neuritis

Optic Neuritis is a condition caused by a temporary swelling from inflammation of the optic nerve. When experiencing optic neuritis, the worst-case scenario is that less blood will flow to the optic nerve; because of poor blood flow, there will be ischemia of the nerve, a part of which could degenerate and wither.

In most cases, optic neuritis comes and goes. Physicians believe they can help this condition with steroid treatments. Sometimes, the steroid treatments work and the optic neuritis does not return frequently. At other times, however, they create dependency.

When you suffer from optic neuritis, a good thing to do is to spend a lot of time in a completely dark room. This gives your whole body, as well as your eyes, a great chance to relax. By far the best solution for optic neuritis is a long session of palming. This is true whether the cause is the optic nerve itself or a systemic illness like multiple sclerosis that impacts many other nerves besides the optic nerve.

Imagine that you walk a lot and step on your legs in an imbalanced way. Consequently, you develop swelling in your legs. Physicians would correctly tell you to rest your leg, maybe to put a brace or a bandage on your ankle, or perhaps to use crutches. Any of the these actions would be to give your leg the rest it needs to heal so that it can return to its proper functioning. In many ways, the same approach is appropriate for the optic nerve. You must rest your optic nerve for the inflammation of the nerve to disappear.

Staying in a dark room, covering your eyes with a light cloth for a day, or perhaps two days, and not walking much in daylight could be the best solution for optic neuritis. It's also good to massage your neck and your back.

This is a very important piece of information for millions of people. No one gives you the suggestion to lie and rest in the dark. Hospital rooms are fully lit all the time for the purpose of security and control. Lack of darkness in many hospital rooms is the reason why a problem like this can be exacerbated. Being at home in the most familiar surroundings can make a difference, especially with fresh air and loving palms over your closed eyes to give you a sense of nurturing. When you lie in the dark with your eyes closed, or when you sit in the dark and palm, you allow for complete replenishment of the optic nerve, which is more important than any medication you can possibly get.

In extreme cases, medication helps. Sometimes, though, medication produces terrible side effects. Sitting in the dark has helped the majority of my clients who have had different attacks of optic neuritis. I advise the clients with whom I work in person that only if this doesn't work should medication become an option. Since you, the reader, are not working with me in person, I advise you to work with a physician who is not opposed to your self-healing practices. Be sure, as you follow my recommendations, to consult with a trusted physician, one who knows your condition well and to whom you have easy access during this process. This will determine the urgency, or not, for you to be put on medication.

When the optic neuritis passes, diligently practice the ten exercises in chapter 2 as well as the previous exercises for unusual nerve phenomena. Also, practice the exercise of throwing the glowing ball in the dark and sunning, along with everything else used for correcting glaucoma.

Correcting Optic Nerve Damage

Most people believe in the absolute determination of extreme conditions; for example, if you are blind, you will never again be able to see. That seems to be your destiny. Nevertheless, there are cases that disprove this notion, and one in particular stands out in my mind.

In February 2009, Simone, a middle-aged pediatric dentist, had a terrible traffic accident in Brazil. Though the surgeries for her fractured skull went very well, her optic nerve had been damaged: she seemed to be completely blind in her right eye and was 97 percent blind in her left eye. She took my six-day course and several individual sessions.

At first, all Simone could see was the first two lines of the Snellen chart from three feet away. Sônia, who worked with me on Simone, was used to seeing many people whose vision was diminished, but it was still difficult to watch a person go from 20/20 to seeing so little in just a few months. In fact, I also find it difficult to see people lose the function of their eyes. Sometimes we have to deal with it as therapists, but it's difficult nonetheless.

I immediately started to treat Simone with eye exercises: sunning, where she closed her eyes and moved her head from side to side while facing the sun, to strengthen her pupils; palming, where she would rub her hands and put them gently over her eye orbits to relax and energize them. Then I patched her left eye, put her in a dark room, and used a blinking light that she was able to see. After that, I took her outdoors and waved a white piece of paper in front of her that reflected the sun; she was not able to see the paper, but she was able to sense its movement. Simone wasn't able to see the paper, nor could she see the strong light of the sun reflecting from the paper, but she could sense from her stronger side when the reflection disappeared. We played a game where she tried to take the paper out of my hand, and she succeeded very quickly. We did it many times. After removing the patch from her left eye, she was able to see four more lines on the chart from the same distance of three feet.

Eventually, Simone traveled with her family all the way to San Francisco to work with me at the School for Self-Healing, where we spent hours together daily. Despite a language difference, because my Portuguese was broken, we understood each other very well. First, I treated her in a dark room; then I massaged Simone's face, had her bounce on a trampoline, and took her to the beach to have her look at the waves. I also patched her left eye and activated her right eye, which seemed at first to have absolutely no vision. One of the biggest accomplishments was that the blinking lights became much clearer, and she was even able to see some shadows and shapes with her blind right eye. The work in the dark room with steam and a cold towel, the love of her husband, who helped me massage her, and the warmth of my good friend Jan, who also helped me work on Simone, not only melted the skepticism of her daughter but also gave Simone a great sense of support—and with that, her healing began.

In January 2010, I met her again in São Paulo, Brazil, and I was surprised at what she saw: 90 percent of normal vision with pinhole glasses. Two years later, I was struggling with the idea of having a root canal; even after five dentists—including some of my students—pressured me to have it done, I still didn't want to do it. So I decided to confide in Simone, as I trusted her completely. At that point, I had not spoken with her for an entire year, but called her long distance anyway. She suggested that I have the root canal, so I went ahead and had it done. Then she told me, "Meir, you gave me my life back. I'm practicing dentistry, and I'm teaching pediatric dentistry at the university. Also, I got my driver's license back."

Despite the fact that physicians had pronounced her incurable, Simone was ultimately able to see again. This was greatly due to our wonderful rapport, but also partly because of her commitment to travel far just to make that connection, regardless of language barriers; the support of her husband didn't hurt either. Interestingly, Simone's daughter—who at first had reservations about my work—decided to study ophthalmology so that she could combine it with self-healing and refer people to practitioners of my work. This was just one unexpected result when someone who used to see only 3 percent of normal vision now sees 97 percent, and who used to walk supported by her husband and daughter now drives to the university on her own. It proved to everyone that a deep connection will not only produce the desired outcome but can also lead to innovation.

Another extraordinary case happened during a visit to Mexico, where I had a small vision class with twelve people, some of whom suffered from normal farsightedness, for which I taught them the principles of natural vision improvement. To their amazement, they started to see well and could even read letters for the first time without wearing glasses. I discovered that three women in the class were blind in one eye, so I patched their seeing eyes and placed blinking lights in front of their blind eyes. The dynamic of the class was that we kept working on vision improvement. And because three of the women were each blind in one eye, I sent them with my two apprentices, Patricia and Laura, to practice the exercises that have been described. Two of the subjects saw it as an exercise and received it pretty well, but one of them cried hysterically because it had prevented her from seeing; she left the room and, half an hour later, returned to the class to work on her presbyopia. The one who cried was named Esperanza, and I met her two days later for a series of three sessions.

When she came for the first session, I asked her, "Esperanza, why did you cry hysterically when Patricia and Laura worked with you in the dark room?" She hugged me and cried, saying, "Meir, when I was seventeen, my father died from an accident. And when my right eye was patched, I felt that sense of loss; it brought it all back." I hugged and kissed her, and then she went to the treatment table. We massaged her face, and put cold and warm towels on it. My apprentices, Patricia and Laura, helped me work with her, and we measured the vision of her left eye; it was perfect. We patched the left eye; with her afflicted right eye, she could not even see the large E on the chart from one foot, which is one-twentieth of the normal distance. Instead she saw a black spot. We took her into a dark room where we used blinking lights. She could see them, but only on one side. We covered that side with the paper, and with the light blinking in the left nasal area of the right eye, she started to see the lights. When we took the patch off, she felt that her vision system had improved. She had the feeling that more light was coming to her eye.

In the next session, we started sunning. As she faced the sun, the pupil would constrict, and as she moved her head away, her pupils would expand. We patched her left eye again and she was able to see the first three lines of the eye chart from two feet. My apprentices and I were amazed and were in awe of the event.

In the last session, we used the Melissa, a strip of paper taped from her forehead to her chin. She threw a ball from hand to hand above her head and was able to catch the ball with her right hand. When we took the Melissa paper off, she felt that she could see better with both eyes. When we finished, Esperanza said to me, "Right now I feel like I got my best forty-sixth birthday gift, because my retina was torn in six different pieces, and no doctor thought I would even see light through it. But now I have peripheral vision with my right eye, and I feel that I'm a safer driver."

She liked the rest of my work because her presbyopia (farsightedness) had improved in her seeing eye, and she could see well from near. As we worked, we discovered that on the right side of her blind eye, even while her strong eye was patched, she could actually see blinking lights. This made no sense because there had been six botched surgeries on her, and any physician would say there was no way she could ever see; however, we were curious enough to find out if there was. After all, Esperanza had come from Bogotá, Columbia, to Cuernavaca, Mexico, in order to work with me. Since she could see from her side, though not from near her nose, I first gave her the blinking exercise: I got her to hold two small blinkers of light; she would look at one, cover it, and then she'd look at the other and cover it. Next, while her strong eye was patched, I also patched the left side of her left eye. When Esperanza blinked her eyes at the nasal area, which she couldn't see before, she started to see that as well. I always teach that legally blind people first have to have a sense of the picture in order to clarify it in the brain and then be able to see it. The beginning of the transition is basically moving from total lack of vision to sensing blinking lights in the darkest possible room.

On the first day, Esperanza had not been able to see the large letter of the eye chart from a foot and a half; if you can't see that letter from twenty feet, then you're considered legally blind. Though she had not seen that letter with her left eye, she still saw that the page was white and that something was interfering with the white. On the second day, she did the sunning exercise: Esperanza closed her eyes and moved her head from side to side. As she faced the sun, her pupils would constrict; when she moved away from it, they would expand and relax. After that, when I patched her right eye, she was able to read the first three lines of the eye chart without any difficulty. Because this attempt was only from a foot and a half away, she was still considered legally blind; however, Esperanza was now sighted.

I situated her in a dark room, put a cold towel over her eyes, and massaged her; my two apprentices massaged her body, while I massaged around her eyes and neck, bringing blood into her head.

When Esperanza was about to return to Columbia, she told me that for several years she had believed she'd never be able to see from her left eye. This is one of the strongest cases I ever had, where, in four days, a woman who was blind for four years was finally able to see—without medication or surgery, but with exercise and massage.

Correcting Detached Retinas and Retinal Tears

A detached retina is a very serious problem that almost always causes partial or full blindness unless it is treated.

The retina performs a function similar to the film in a camera. Located in the back of the eye, it receives optical images, converts them to chemical reactions, and transmits them through the optic nerve to the brain for interpretation.

The retina is considered to be detached whenever it is removed from its normal position in the back of the eye. This can occur in anybody at any age. People who are experiencing retinal detachment report seeing "floaters" (dark spots that seem to move around in their field of vision) or a gray curtain moving back and forth across their eyes.

There are many reasons for detached retinas. The most familiar ones are myopia—mainly high myopia, when the eyeball is very long—as well as post-cataract surgeries and traumas. Blows to the head can also create retinal detachments. In my opinion, this is another reason to avoid LASIK surgery, since it weakens the eye, creating greater chances of a retinal detachment simply by bumping your head forcefully.

If the retinal detachment is very large, you must see a physician soon, because the detachment can cause lack of blood flow to the photoreceptors and can kill them. Within a short period of time, possibly a week or two, you can lose your vision. As an exception, I met a person who had a violent fight in prison, during which he received a head-butt. As a result of the fight, his retina detached and the prison physician was not capable of diagnosing it. After he had served his term, he was seen by a top ophthalmologist, who told him that he had already had a detachment for several months. He had reattachment surgery and, to his amazement, as well as his ophthalmologist's and my own, his vision returned almost to normal, and the retina was functional. But this is extraordinary, and most of the time it doesn't happen that way. Usually, within a couple of weeks of lack of blood flow to the photoreceptors, they die. What should we do then?

A female patient came to me once, complaining of a retinal detachment in one eye and poor vision in the other. One thing I noticed was that she wasn't blinking. She told me it was written in her medical chart that she wasn't blinking, but none of her doctors had paid attention to the notation. Therefore, I told her to blink, and her vision improved very quickly after that.

Pay attention to your demeanor. Are you blinking? Are you not blinking? Do you pay attention to your retina or not? Also, when you have a retinal detachment, make sure that you don't bend your head, or the retina can fall even more. After the healing process, it's important for you to get a lot of massage on your neck and on your back, in order to bring more blood to the head and to strengthen your retina with nurturing blood flow to the eyes. But some of the exercises for loosening your neck (for example, in the section on glaucoma) could hurt, since they require you to bend your head down, which could cause damage. In the acute time of retinal detachment, don't do movement exercises; instead, massage is the best option to relax the tension in your neck and back. After the detachment has healed, it's okay to return to the movement exercises.

Some of the reasons for retinal detachment are emotional. A boy I once knew told me that, after his retinal reattachment surgery, he woke up after the surgery and discovered he had some vision. But, because his mother was not in the room, it traumatized him and he became blind again. There are tissues that respond to our emotions, so it's important to be as calm as you can be, even in the hardest of situations. It can preserve both your sanity and your retina.

Exercise Program for Retinal Detachment

Look at Details (with the parts of your eyes that are not functioning well, by covering the parts that do see well): 10 minutes daily.

Look into the Distance: 40 minutes daily, in 10-minute intervals.

Palming: 24 minutes daily, 6 minutes at a time (once a week, as long as you do not have glaucoma, sit down and palm for an hour, listening to something pleasant like music or a book on tape).

Darkness and Light Exercise: 20 minutes daily.

With retinal detachment, after exercising the blind or the fuzzy spot, quite a few people start to have some more vision in it, which is a wonderful phenomenon. It happens because some of the cells are only dormant, even though some are dead. So, when we wake up the dormant cells, we have access to more vision.

Figure 6.11. Look at the details with the parts of your eyes that are not functioning well.

Extra Exercise for Retinal Detachment: Darkness and Light

If parts of your retina are dead, or if you have a sighted eye, patch your sighted eye and obstruct the parts of your disabled eye that are still functioning with paper. Then look at the world through holes in the paper, using only the parts of your eyes that do not function well.

Four times a day, after six minutes of palming, go into a closed room and use blinking lights. At the School for Self-Healing we sell small

Figure 6.12. Use blinking or flashing lights in a dark room to activate the parts of the eyes that are not working.

Figure 6.13. The small blinking lights we use at the school.

Figure 6.14. Our magic wands.

blinking lights you can use for this exercise, but any different-colored blinking lights will do. The object is simply to turn on the blinking lights to activate the parts of your eyes that are not working.

When you have the functional parts of your eyes covered and you are looking at blinking lights in a dark room, you may not see anything at all at first, but over time you may start to see small changes in the darkness. Small flashes of light may start to occur. Be patient. In time you may start to see more and more flashing lights and, eventually, shapes may start to occur. Sometimes a picture comes; when it does, it's wonderful.

A much more subtle way of accomplishing this same exercise is to obstruct the functional part of your eyes, and walk outside in bright sunlight, crossing between a brightly lit area and a shaded area. Walk with somebody who can help you to make sure you do not trip. Move your head from side to side, but do not move your eyes. Look up at the sky, where you can see the light of the sun and the sky, and look down at the shade, where you may be able to see that it is darker, and that distinction may start to give you a sense of contrast. The extremes of light and dark may start to become apparent over time. In this way, you are accomplishing the same thing as with the blinking lights. You are activating the part of your eyes that does not function well, so that vision in your blind spot will start to develop.

If you have some vision, obstruct the sighted area in your eyes with a patch over the strong eye, and paper with cut-out holes for the weak areas to look through, over the weak eye. Now walk in your garden or somewhere safe, with a companion who can hold your hand or catch you if you fall, and move your head from side to side slowly so as to help you notice more details. Then take off your patches; 75 percent of people who do this see an immediate improvement in their vision. The improvement is temporary, but repetition of this exercise makes it become stable.

Correcting Vitreous Detachment

The vitreous is what we call the gel-like substance between the retina and the lens, and it is in fact attached to the retina via millions of fine, intertwined fibers. As the vitreous shrinks from age and neglect, detachment from the retina can occur.

Vitreous detachment is much more common, but less harmful, than retinal detachment. Only in rare cases does vitreous detachment lead to partial blindness. But it does lead to a tremendous amount of floaters that obstruct vision. A floater is what we call a tiny dark spot that seems to be "floating" around in your field of vision, obstructing what you are looking at.

In a minority of cases, vitreous detachment can lead to retinal detachment or puckers, by pulling apart the retina; this, in turn, can lead to bleeding and flooding of the photoreceptor cells, causing blindness. But most of the time, it's relatively harmless and just leads to some floaters.

Normally, with a retinal pucker, after looking at an eye chart and seeing it to some extent, there is a sense of clarity in the rest of your visual system. If you take off the patch, you will find that your vision is very much clearer. That's why repetition of these exercises is so useful.

If you experience vitreous detachment, however, I recommend getting checked by two or three ophthalmologists, especially retinal specialists, to be sure that the detachment didn't cause any harm to the retina at the same time.

Often, people are afraid of the floaters. A good way to deal with them might seem rather amazing and unpredictable. The secret is, you look at them. You just walk outdoors on a sunny day, or at least on a bright day, and look at the floaters one by one. If you cannot see them one by one because there are groups of floaters, look at them group by group. When you isolate and look at the floaters, you cause the vitreous fluid to collide against the floaters, which breaks them up and causes them to disappear.

For example, if you have more floaters in your right eye, patch or obstruct your left eye, and walk for twenty minutes in the sun, with a nice view to look at. As you look at the view, floaters will appear. As they appear, look right at the floaters and, as you do, the vitreous fluid will collide against them and destroy them. Normally, what happens when you look at a floater, is that it floats away, then it comes back; when you look at it again, your vitreous fluid hits the floater and breaks it into pieces. Then you see smaller pieces, and you look at either one of them or at several pieces, and you break them once again.

Look at a floater that you choose to look at, possibly the larger one, and when the floater floats away, look into the distance. Then look at that floater again when it comes back, and exercise with that floater, back and forth, every day. Most likely, after a few weeks, that floater will disappear. Then you choose the next one. Do it in a neutral state of mind, blink, and breathe. If you have floaters in both eyes, but more in

one eye than the other, patch the eye with fewer floaters and look at the
floaters with the other eye.

I had a patient named Tony who had laser surgeries, retinal detachment, and terrible vitreous floaters. Moreover, he couldn't drive. His doctor had unfortunately told him to wear sunglasses. That only made the
floaters worse. I told him to do a lot of sunning, to walk, and to look at
the floaters. I will never forget the time I walked with him up and down
a hill around my previous office. He looked at plants, he looked at the
view, and very quickly, he improved his vision from 20/200 with glasses
to 20/20 with glasses; he also reduced his diopter level significantly, from
13 to 8 diopters.

Tony reduced his myopia and reduced the floaters, and his vision
became much better compared to how it was; it is better without his
glasses and it's better with his glasses, and with much less correction.
(This wonderful man volunteered to be the model on my DVD, *Yoga for
your Eyes,* which has helped many people to see better.)

Tony used the internal forces in his own body to improve his eyes, and
the improvement was massive. So can you. Your internal forces are only
partially known, and they're stronger than what anyone can imagine.

Even though many floaters are not a result of vitreous detachment,
the treatment is the same. You have to mentally accept the fact that it's
okay for you to have this floater; then you have to look at it. If you've
lived with floaters for many years and it's familiar to you, it will probably
be hard for your mind to believe they can disappear. If it is one floater,
look at it. If there are groups of floaters, look only at one group. If it
is a big floater, look at one part of it. Repeated exercises will show you
that you can actually decrease it, change its shape and, with time, rid
yourself of it. The only thing that keeps the floater going is your disgust
for that floater and lack of willingness to look at it. That's what happens
with most people. We have forces within us that can destroy that which
impedes us, if we only let them do it.

Additionally, what we learn from the fact that we are experiencing
vitreous detachment in the first place is that the health of the eye is going
in the wrong direction. Therefore, once we eliminate the floaters, we must

return to the basic eye exercises in the beginning of this book in order to strengthen and heal the entire eye.

Correcting Macular Puckers and Holes

Some people suddenly discover they can no longer see centrally. It's a scary situation. From the person's viewpoint, one day he or she sees perfectly, and the next day the central vision has disappeared. When the person meets an ophthalmologist, the ophthalmologist has absolutely nothing to offer that person except sympathy.

Often, this situation is caused by macular holes and macular puckers—basically, detachment of the vitreous that takes with it a part of the macula. Other times, we simply have cells that have withered and died. In all cases, the treatment is the same.

Exercise Program for Macular Holes and Puckers:
80 Minutes a Day

Palming: 24 minutes daily, 6 minutes at a time.
Sunning: 30 minutes daily, in three 10-minute intervals.
Skying (if there is no sun): 8 minutes daily.
Long Swing: 5 minutes daily.
Extra Exercise: Pinhole Glasses: 10 minutes daily.

Figure 6.15. Pinhole glasses and pinhole glasses with obstruction.

Remember not to simply take one part of the day and do your eye exercises all at once. The best results come from working on your eyes all the time, throughout your day. Find a few minutes here and there, and let the eye exercises in this book find their way naturally into your routine. Thus, vision improvement will be created in an organic way in your daily life. This is the way to improve for the long term.

Extra Pinhole Glasses Exercise

Pinhole glasses are opaque glasses with many tiny holes punched through the lenses.

Put the pinhole glasses on, then cover the eye that sees normally. Use the eye that has the macular hole in it to look straight ahead at an eye chart. You should put the eye chart in full light or, if there is sun, in full sunlight. The pinhole glasses will protect you from the temporary glare, and your tendency will be to tilt your head to see. Don't tilt your head; instead, look straight ahead. Then close your eyes and remember exactly how the letters looked to you.

At times, you will only see the very big letter from a very short distance. If that's what you see, it's okay. Allow that area of your eye to be functional. After you remember the exact shape and contour of the letter or letters that you saw, open your eyes and look again.

Now move your head very slightly from side to side, less than a quarter of an inch. That's enough for you to see the letter moving in the opposite direction than the way *you* are moving, through the fuzz or the veil that you are looking through.

The next step is to put masking tape on the pinhole lens covering the area that would be the central periphery, and do the same exercise.

Normally, when you have a macular pucker, you see better peripherally. So, next, cover the entire weaker lens with construction paper that has only a tiny hole, made by a pen or pencil right where the main blind spot is in your vision. Now look at the eye chart through that pinhole you made.

Note: It is dangerous to create a hole in the paper while you are wearing these glasses. Do not create the hole while the paper is on your face. Even though it seems easiest to do it this way (since only then can you test

Figure 6.16. Use the eye that has the macular hole in it to look straight ahead at an eye chart.

whether or not the hole is in the correct spot), it is best to find the blind spot and to create the hole on the paper when it is away from your eyes. It may take you a few tries until the hole is positioned right in front of the fuzzy or blind spot, but do not do it in front of your face, even if it seems more convenient to do so.

Sometimes it's impossible to see any print through the hole. If that is the case with your vision, you should start this exercise by stimulating that area with blinking lights, like the ones you can order through our School for Self-Healing in San Francisco.

With a macular pucker, some cells are still alive, but they are dormant in most cases, and they're not being activated. Looking at the eye chart, only with the fuzzy area in your central field, will clarify your vision. Even slight clarification can make a big difference to your visual system because it eases the burden on the rest of the cells.

Correcting Retinitis Pigmentosa

Retinitis pigmentosa is an inherited disease characterized by a gradual, progressive degeneration of the retina. This leads to loss of peripheral vision and night vision difficulties, and can also lead to central vision loss as well.

If you know that you are predisposed to retinitis pigmentosa, you should start to work on shifting and peripheral vision exercises at a very young age. If you do this, you would simply be diagnosed as having some missing spots in your visual system, but you would basically see well.

Although retinitis pigmentosa is genetic in nature, it is exacerbated by the normal stresses in life. What are our stresses? It is stressful when you look at someone and can see only their head and not the rest of them. It is even more stressful to see everything fuzzy. Another major source of stress is caused by the vision loss itself. It is especially stressful when you see well enough to get by, but not well enough to function fully. You may walk on the street and see people, but you don't recognize your friend's face immediately. Mental stress occurs from people having their feelings hurt by that, and from you criticizing yourself about it, even though you would forgive anyone else for not being able to see someone's face.

I think it's very important to announce to the world, "I do have an eye disease and, if you want me to recognize you, just say, 'Here I am.' Sometimes don't say it, see if I recognize you first, and only if I don't, then say, 'Here I am.' And if I do recognize you, that's a great thing. I'm seeing you, and you acknowledged that."

Let people know that there is suffering involved in your life, and don't have them feel bad or guilty about it. You'd be amazed how much people's intelligence grows when they understand how to treat other people, and how much it shrinks when you hide a phenomenon that you are experiencing.

From the very first year that I had started to work on overcoming my blindness while also working on others, I found out that those people who hide a serious problem always suffer for it. Even if they have a good reason to hide (for example, because they would be fired from work), at the end of the day, they still suffer more from hiding than from revealing it.

Other people revere their problems and use them as a crutch or as a tool to gain favors; they try to get others to do special things for them that they wouldn't have done had they not known of a problem. Those people don't heal either.

The people who heal are the ones who look at the problem as a matter of fact. I could be short, I could be tall, I could have cataracts, I could have retinitis pigmentosa, I could limp; either way, I'm a whole person, I'm okay, and I just have to deal with my problems as well as my triumphs. The problem becomes much less of a problem when it's being discussed.

Exercise Program for Retinitis Pigmentosa

Note: You should not start this book with the section on retinitis pigmentosa. If you did, go back to the beginning of the book and work from the Introduction on. Be aware of all the deep concepts of life, vitality, and vision. Then you will be ready to work with this chapter.

Palming: 24 minutes daily.
Sunning: 20 minutes daily.
Night Walking: One hour, twice a week (if possible).
Shifting: 10 minutes daily.
Extra Exercise for Retinitis Pigmentosa: 20 minutes daily.

A Note about Night Walking

Sometimes night walking is not possible because your vision is not strong enough in the dark. In this case, you cannot walk at night. The ability to night walk could come as a result of improvement in your peripheral vision.

There's a big difference between simply sitting in a dark room and actually walking around in the dark. The body is meant to respond to visual information, therefore the brain receives the impulses much better through movement in the dark than through being still.

If your vision isn't clear enough at night, because so many people with retinitis pigmentosa lose that capacity, you may still see well enough to adapt to your room with some light from the outside. In that case, spend about an hour each night for the next six months exercising in the following sequence: first walk back and forth in your room; then sit cross-legged on the floor (occasionally moving in a rotating motion just enough to create the sensation of movement); finally, walk forward and backward again. This should begin to stimulate some cells that are just dormant and not dead. If you do that, there's a good chance you will slow down the retinitis pigmentosa greatly, and eventually develop good enough night vision to go night walking.

I will never forget the person in his forties who came to me with retinitis pigmentosa. His mother had lost her vision to retinitis pigmentosa, the same way he did. His vision was very clear when he looked at an eye chart: it was 20/30 with his glasses on, which was within the normal range; peripherally, he didn't even have 3 percent vision. Whenever he would step to a slightly darker room, not even completely dark, but just slightly darker, he would be blind momentarily. So I taught him to palm for fifteen seconds whenever he stepped into a dark room. When he took his hands from his eyes, he saw much better.

In order to improve his peripheral vision, we created an exercise that required three assistants but ended up being very successful. Remember that the periphery senses movement, and the central vision mainly senses a still picture. The exercise we created made use of this principle in a dynamic way. I had one assistant stand in front of the patient and throw a ball back and forth to him. While they played catch, I had two more assistants stand on either side of the man, throwing a ball back and forth across his field of vision. The tennis balls were crossing each other in the backyard. Slowly, he started to notice the ball going side to side more and more. It was gradual, but he was becoming more aware of the periphery.

After four days of intensive training, his peripheral vision improved to 85 percent. There's no question that, even though the treatment was very intensive and fruitful, the therapy did not regenerate 80 percent to 82 percent of his peripheral field in four days. In all likelihood, what had happened was that, although many cells had already died, most others were simply dormant and, by doing the work that we did, we woke up the dormant cells, thus helping him to regain and to maintain his vision for many years. Later that year, he reported to us that he no longer bumped his head against airplane compartments, and that he was able to see when hands were raised by kids in his classes. It turns out he was Superintendent of Education for the State of Michigan, and whenever he had gone to class in the past, when he looked straight ahead, he wouldn't see anyone who had raised a hand. Now he could.

So whenever you move to a more dimly lit room, palm at most for forty-five seconds. Put your hands over your eye orbits and visualize that you're seeing darkness, or maybe even blackness. Breathe deeply and slowly. The breathing will bring you oxygen and relaxation. The palming will widen your pupils and will allow the healthy cells in your retina to function better. Then you will find that the room becomes clearer.

Extra Exercises for Retinitis Pigmentosa:
The Mask of Zorro

The majority of people with retinitis pigmentosa lose their peripheral vision, but for a while keep their central vision. A minority of people with retinitis pigmentosa just see better peripherally and worse centrally. Other people lose their vision almost completely. In each case, it's very important for us to work on ourselves, confronting our own personal manifestation of the problem, patiently and frequently.

If you lost most of your central vision to retinitis pigmentosa, place construction paper, with a hole poked out in the area of your central vision, over your eye. Walk in daylight, whether in the garden or in the street, with someone who will hold your hand, unless you're independent enough. Even though you blocked the vision that you are using most of the time, observe all the details that you can see. Look at smaller details than the ones that you can easily see. So, on the one hand, you would say, "I already have a much smaller portion of the picture." But, at the same time, you want to build a sense of central vision. Central vision is such that we always look at smaller details than the ones we see.

Look at smaller and smaller details and you will start to see them better and better. Walk with the paper on your eye for a minimum of forty minutes a day, and a maximum of one hundred minutes a day. At first, you may not be able to tolerate the paper for more than ten minutes at a time; in that case, do it eight minutes at a time, and never strain. Always palm before you do it, sometimes palm in the middle of doing it, and often palm after you finish walking with the obstructive construction paper that does not let you see the periphery. Look straight ahead.

Some people laughingly call this exercise "The Mask of Zorro." Walk with the Mask of Zorro and observe all the details you can see through it.

What you're giving yourself is a chance to wake up all the dormant cells in the center of your retina.

One thing you need to remember is that memory is a powerful tool. Whatever you look at, as fuzzy as it may appear (due to the cells that were destroyed), if you close your eyes and remember it exactly how it was seen, when you open your eyes, it will be at least a tad clearer, and sometimes much more so.

After a few weeks of closing your eyes and remembering what you saw, close your eyes and remember contrast. If you look at white flowers versus green leaves, close your eyes and say, "The flowers are white; the leaves are green," and in your mind, visualize the flowers to be even brighter white and the leaves to be even darker green. In addition, you could visualize greater sharpness of the different colors that you saw. You could look at the sky and say, "The sky is bright blue and the clouds are white." To create as much contrast as you could, close your eyes and say, "The ocean is blue, and the waves are white." The imagery has to come with a sense of realistic colors.

Then visualize larger objects. Visualize that the petals of a flower are large and distinct, even though they may look small, or almost nonexistent with the poor vision you have. Visualize a greater amount of details than the amount of details that you saw with your eyes open.

When you look with the area that is nearly blind, the most important thing is to look through it as if that's all you can see with. Many people are very disturbed with the whole concept of looking with an area that is damaged. But that's where healing begins: where you accept exactly the space that you are in. Nurturing your weakest area and feeling okay with it will strengthen every part of your life. You will take away the pressure on the rest of your visual system, and it will be easier for you to use your eyes. Parts of your brain that are no longer active, because of a lack of stimuli from the exact blind spots, will start to work.

You will gain back some of the normal vision in the blind spot. Sometimes the blind spot decreases, and you can slowly control and manage your vision. The loss you would have experienced over a period of five years stretches to a period of twenty-five years, and your visual life becomes more normal and more predictable.

Waving Lights in the Dark

If walking outside in the starlight or in the moonlight is way too difficult and above your capacity, but your central vision is good or even excellent, then sit in a dark room and turn the lights on and off. We also have large glow sticks, which are plastic wands that light up gently in many different colors and blink. The good thing about the wands—we call them magic wands—is that when you wave them at the side of your head, on both sides, as you look straight ahead, they stimulate your peripheral vision.

If you darken the room, use a room that has no windows, or if you put heavy curtains on your windows, and you wave either the wand light or a candle in the dark, the movement will wake up many of the dormant cells that you have. The benefit of the flame of a candle is that it moves, and the movement of the flame activates the rods of the retina. What's good about wand lights is that you can wave them. Also, they have stronger light than candles and they don't drip wax. Sometimes the wand lights are too strong for the eyes to exercise and improve as compared to candles.

Spending positive time with your eyes will eliminate the negativity you hear about or experience with them. I once had a patient who came to me in San Francisco from Australia. She was able to improve her central vision from nearsightedness to nearly normal vision, and did not need glasses to look straight ahead, but she had severe retinitis pigmentosa. For ten years, she did not walk freely outdoors at night, but she did walk freely outdoors in the daytime. After she practiced waving lights in the dark, and also having extensive amounts of massage, she was able to walk at night on dark streets for the first time.

For the first few weeks of this exercise, do not use the pieces of paper taped to the bridge of your nose. Then gradually start to use the small, medium, and large pieces of paper taped to the bridge of your nose. Wave the wand lights to the sides of your eyes, and you may get a sense that one eye sees more light than the other eye. If this is the case, close the eye that sees more light for a short while—about five or six seconds—and only use the other eye; then open both eyes and use both. The idea is to create evenness between the two eyes and to make the brain immediately use peripheral vision.

Sometimes, the wand lights will not be visible. Other times, people with retinitis pigmentosa will not notice the color of the lights. So it is better to start with red blinking lights because red has the longest wavelengths, making it the easiest light to see. Then, over time, you can change to different colors.

Truly, anytime someone is experiencing a blind spot, blinking lights and wand lights in a dark room can bring to life the parts of the eye that are not functioning. In this way, you start to create that process of slowly expanding that which you are capable of doing.

A Final Note about Peripheral Exercises

When you have retinitis pigmentosa, no matter what condition your eyes are in, make it a habit to notice the periphery throughout the day. Work the periphery every waking moment. For a few seconds at a time, do the waving of hands in your periphery throughout the day. This way, the two eyes are working together. In the center, one eye can dominate; with the periphery, however, both eyes must work, so one eye cannot dominate the other.

When you wave your hands quickly to the sides of your eyes and close one eye, you only see one hand waving. Close the other eye and you only see the other hand waving. Open both eyes and you see both hands waving. This way you know that both eyes are working together. Go back to chapter 2 and focus mainly on the ten steps.

Chapter 7

Working with Children

We need to learn how to work with our children with the ten steps in chapter 2. I want to refer to how I've worked with my own daughter, using the balls that were far away from each other and then getting closer and closer. What's amazing with my daughter is how well she sees without glasses—sometimes as well as 20/50, even 20/40, which is 80 percent of 20/20. Even these days, when my daughter—who's already twenty-three—is being tested by a regular optometrist who simply is stressed and sees her like any other client, or gets a little bit nervous about her condition, as she has no lens—it's called an aphakic eye, and she has a small cornea called microphthalmia—she sees worse. For example, when my daughter went to a new optometrist near a university where she studied in DC, he measured her vision as 20/70 with contact lenses, and she was embarrassed. She didn't even want to show me the results because I had measured her vision as 20/20 at times. Then, here in San Francisco, she was sent to another optometrist who spoke in a way that made sense to her. She complained that her eyes get dry, so he asked her, "Do you drink coffee?" When she said yes, he told her that drinking coffee dries her eyes. He looked at her acidity level and determined she was too acidic. Then he told her that he did not believe in doctors and tried not to go to them himself. Because of her background and her feeling about doctors—although she loved her pediatric ophthalmologist and her pediatrician, and liked many doctors in general—her philosophy is the same: it's holistic; you don't just allow people to push medicines on you. She felt at home with this particular optometrist, and when he fitted her with contact lenses, her vision was nearly 20/25: almost 95 percent of 20/20. The assumption is that if you see with contacts less than 20/20, you will still see 20/20 or better with glasses. It was very interesting that even at the age of twenty-two—not a child any more, but a young adult—when she met a good optometrist, and one to whom she could relate, her vision got much better. I was told by some of my student optometrists that when they massaged children's shoulders, with the same prescription those children could see two or three lines better on the eye chart; but to jump from 20/70 to 20/25 is to jump by 5 lines on the chart, and that comes only when you're completely relaxed. Normally, as I mentioned before, when someone has cataracts and the lens is removed, they need glass lenses because glasses help you to see better than contacts. On the contrary, in the case of nearsightedness, contacts allow you to see better than glasses. And children who don't have a lens replacement see much better through thick glasses.

Kids have to be played with. You can never simply show them exercises and expect them to follow the exercises. Take them to the ocean and show them the waves, patching the strong eye and looking with the weak eye at the waves; play ball with them using an obstructive lens (and to remind you: pop out one lens of cheap sunglasses and put obstructive paper over the other lens), and throw and catch the ball. If your child has blind spots, put him in the dark and cover the area that sees with a patch, then use blinking lights for the area that doesn't see. These lights can be purchased at the School for Self-Healing.

Figure 7.1. If you have a child with one weak eye, it's most important that the child should obstruct the strong eye with small obstruction glasses.

When we work with our young children, it helps for it to take the form of a game. Some examples of this have already been described. The best game form is working with red and green glasses. Another is the one with balls rolling at different distances, starting with a short distance (like half a yard), then going to a yard, to two yards, and so on. We can put two bowls about two feet apart, then get them closer when the ball rolls between them, to a foot and a half apart, and then get them closer to eight inches apart when the ball rolls again. We can do eleven or twelve games that way. If you have a child with one weak eye, it's most important that the child should obstruct the eye—which is even better than patching—with small obstruction glasses.

You can also have the child look at flower petals or at a shifter while looking at black and white stripes, which are basically a nice way of looking up and down on each one of those stripes from beginning to end and vice versa. This will get the child to connect to central vision, to a central fixation. At the same time, it's very important to work on the periphery. A good game for that is to obstruct the strong eye with a small piece of paper, wave your hand to the side of the strong eye, and catch and throw a ball—but it's important that the hand has to keep waving.

When a kid is in his early adolescence, at the age of twelve or thirteen, make sure they are looking far into a distance and playing games after half an hour of computer use. And every time, after half an hour of computer use, have the child go out. There was a story in the Israeli newspapers about a mother who brought her daughter to get glasses. The ophthalmologist asked how long her daughter spent looking at a computer, and the answer was that she did so quite a bit. He advised her that after every half hour, her daughter had to play for half an hour, and glasses would not even be needed. Her vision became better than 20/20.

The same thing is needed for teenagers. One thing I'm seeing with many teenagers and young adults is that they like to go to bed late: 1 a.m. to 3 a.m. is common. And whether you're a younger or an older adult, lights should be out earlier. We should all be sure to get an ample amount of rest. Listen to relaxing music, listen to a nice book on tape, but go to sleep early. Sleeping late leads to continuous fatigue of the body. Also, teenagers should always stretch in the morning and then do all the exercises in the section on myopia in chapter 4. It will work for them just fine, but it's important to interest them as well. They should look at waves with their weaker eye or look at twelve different points on the horizon and then see twelve different points closer and closer, maybe even seeing boats at a distance. They should play ball; throw the teenager a ball and then kick it, maybe playing with three people together.

If a parent is working with their kid, the parent should do the same thing. That's the only way that the kid will do it as well. For example, if you want your kid to work on his nearsightedness, work on your near-sightedness. If you want them to patch their stronger eye, patch your own stronger eye or use obstructive lenses. If you want them to look into the distance, do it yourself. The more you do it, the more you believe in it because you will see the results, and your belief will radiate to your kids. Again, playing ball and working at all angles will improve their field of vision. It would also be helpful to work on the peripheral exercises that we mentioned previously.

Years ago, Melissa, whom I talk about in this book, was a patient of Dr. Creig Hoyt, professor of ophthalmology at the University of California, San Francisco, School of Medicine, and he was very impressed with the improvement she had made using our method. Because he was also impressed with other clients of mine, and because of his experience with my children, and because of his stature—at the time he was considered one of the top pediatric ophthalmologists in the world—Melissa asked him to write a letter recommending research be done on our work. This marvelous man has done just that.

We have no means to discover how one goes about doing this research; neither do we have financial means, nor do we have the personnel. The times that we have contacted the UCSF School of Optometry, the UCSF School of Ophthalmology, and Pacific Presbyterian Hospital—well-known institutions in the Bay area—we always had a warm reception, but they never sent us people to research our work.

Thus far, ten optometrists, ophthalmologists, and vision profes-sionals have written wonderful acknowledgements, giving us tremen-dous endorsement, but we are still looking for others who will continue researching our work. I hope this quote by a top ophthalmologist will convince more medical professionals of the value that additional research could have for work that will revolutionize the field through natural vision improvement.

The plasticity and potential of the visual system is continuously being explored and redefined. Old notions give way to new potentials. Meir Schneider addresses these issues in his clinical work with patients with various visual problems. His reflections and theories are worth consideration and critical review.

> ■ Creig Hoyt, MD, professor and chair of the ophthalmology department at UCSF Medical School; director of Beckman Vision Center, San Francisco; and editor of the *British Journal of Ophthalmology*. Hoyt is regarded as one of the world's leading pediatric neuro-ophthalmologists. His pioneering studies changed the practice of infant cataract care worldwide.

When we spend a great deal of time focusing on what is directly in front of us, we tend to ignore our peripheral field. To demonstrate the notion that urban life causes atrophy in the perception of peripheral vision, I'd like to present data from a study conducted in Sorocaba, Brazil, whose objective was to assess the effect of visual and physical exercises on visual acuity, based on the Self-Healing Method. The study was developed in four phases and took place over a three-month period, with a group that consisted of thirty-five students in the first to fifth grades, along with two teachers and the preventative purpose of acquiring healthy habits involving vision, body, and breathing. The amazing results reinforce the importance of the evaluation and visual therapy associated with neuropsychomotor development, facilitating learning and socialization of the student:

- In visual acuity, there was an improvement of 39.4 percent in both eyes in reading a line on the Snellen chart from afar.
- In close visual acuity, using the table of large and small letters from the Self-Healing Method, the most significant improvement observed was 24.2 percent in reading letters of type 4 font.
- In relation to the final evaluation of peripheral vision, there was an improvement of 42.8 percent of students who achieved the angle of 90 degrees.

- In the positive results of fusion tests with paper, there was an improvement of 8.6 percent, and on the fusion test with beads, an improvement of 22.8 percent.

This is the first credible research that was done on this work, after so many years of practice. The physical therapists that did this research did it on their own time and were happy to do so. The results were very good. My results are even better with my clients, including children. I would love to have much more research done at the School for Self-Healing and worldwide. If you would like to help us, please donate to the School for Self-Healing. If you have relevant knowledge, donate your knowledge and your time. Or, if possible, you can donate funds for the purpose of researching and saving children's vision and adult vision with the natural therapy we do.

The conclusive data support my belief that many visual problems result from straining to see, read, and write, a bad habit acquired in the first years of school as students try to please parents and teachers. This tension can be alleviated with relaxation techniques as well as physical and visual exercises, leading to improved visual acuity, and learning that will last a lifetime.

Let me give you a couple of examples of what can be done for children. One that illustrates the body's amazing power to heal is about Nancy, an eighteen-year-old indigenous Canadian who had suffered from a thyroid problem that resulted in an undeveloped optic nerve. Her left eye was legally blind: she could see 20/200—which is 20 percent of normal vision—with it, and could read from no farther than two inches; her right eye was completely blind, except for color and light perception.

Nancy's mother had heard about my work and brought her to see me. Our first goal was to stimulate Nancy's weaker eye by completely patching her stronger left eye with thick black paper, all the way from her nose to her temples, and from her forehead to her cheekbone. Then I had her also cover the patched eye with both hands, and in a totally dark room, I turned on a blinking red light. In about a minute, Nancy was able to see exactly where the light came from; a minute later, she was able to see the shape of the light bulb; after another minute, she saw my general features;

two minutes later, she was even able to describe my face. It was a powerful experience that Nancy didn't immediately comprehend because previous clinical tests failed to provide such dramatic results. The reason for this was that they had been conducted too quickly after covering her strong eye and didn't give the brain and nerve pathways enough time to wake up.

With her strong eye still covered, I took Nancy outside for the next exercise: she bounced on a trampoline while throwing and catching large, colorful balls. Though she felt unbalanced, she was nonetheless able to accomplish this using her right eye alone.

For an entire week, we spent daily sessions with Nancy's strong eye patched, walking up and down the street, looking at signs and other objects with her weak eye. When we finally measured, her supposedly blind eye was 20/400 from afar, while her stronger eye improved to 20/60; her vision was closer to normal than it had ever been. If she had not been sitting in that dark room with the blinking light, she would never have known that she had vision in her right eye, and the left eye would never have progressed.

From Nancy's case we discovered that it takes about three to five minutes for a lazy eye to respond, because the brain is suppressing the activity of that eye. When I sat down and chatted with her during our first appointment, her vision had improved from 20/200 to 20/100. Her mother said, "But we went to all the big specialists in Canada, and she never saw that well." I said, "She's comfortable with me because I'm not an uptight physician."

Her mother also realized that she was being overly protective because Nancy had enough vision to bike and to walk, which gave the girl much more freedom. Her mother acknowledged that Nancy saw just as well as her without her glasses. She said, "It's not such bad vision, and I'm way too protective." This is something that is so important for parents to know. One joke that comes to mind is that children wear sweaters when their mothers feel cold. We're so protective of our children that even if they have vision that is manageable, like 50 percent or 60 percent of 20/20, we try to restrict them: we want them to wear glasses, and if glasses don't help, we restrict their activity. Whenever her daughter rode a bicycle, walked, or played sports, Nancy's mother was very afraid for her.

As a result, the daughter had to rebel against her mother. Now, mother and daughter are united. In fact, Nancy's father, who was skeptical at first, was so impressed by the results that he encouraged her to return for treatment, so the entire family made the trip together.

During that visit our emphasis was on eye teaming—getting the two eyes to work together. When she was seeing only with her left eye there was so much pressure on that eye and the whole visual system that her vision was fuzzy. Besides the exercises we did to clarify the vision in her left eye there was great relaxation in seeing with both eyes. By distributing the vision between the two eyes she improved from 20 percent to 70 percent of normal vision. And that's the way to go with children and adults.

Another wonderful story is that one of my students in Brazil called to tell me that her grandson was born with toxoplasmosis—when you have bacteria or a virus sitting in the placenta and it attacks parts of the body after birth, quite often the eye; in this case, it was the right macula, the central, most precious part of the retina, which led to blindness in the right eye. She asked, "Should we just listen to the doctors who said he'll have vision in the left eye, forget the right eye?" I said, "No way." Then I told her to patch his left eye, and have a blinking light in front of his right eye. I said to play with him and use instruments with both sound and light.

In fact, I've seen something from an electric store that made noise and light like a traffic light: green, yellow, and red, blinking on and off and making different noises with each color. I asked them to reproduce that effect. Or simply use a light that blinks with a circuit breaker: 40 watts, or only 15 watts if the infant responds to it; sometimes as many as 60 or 80 watts, depending on if you see that the infant is curious. You can also use the simple, small light that we sell at the school, which blinks as you get close or far from the infant. Then take the infant outdoors with a patch and play games, but only after you did light and dark games in a dark room.

They called me twenty days later, when I returned from an overseas trip, and told me the doctor had said that there was only a small scar in his right eye and that most of the macula functioned. I told them, "Don't stop working with him. Now stimulate the two eyes: patch one eye, and then the other eye, take him outdoors, show him details, and talk to him about all the objects you are showing him in spite of the fact that he's only an infant." What I eventually heard was, "There is no scar. The two eyes see perfectly fine." At the age of four there was another attack, as the virus was still in his nervous system, and so we continued with the exercises. I met him when he reached the age of eight. His father was religious, and they were studying in a religious school, doing much reading, and we had to deal with simple myopia: no obstruction, no disappearance of the central vision; it was simple nearsightedness, corrected with glasses, and we worked on maintaining the clarity of his vision. It was hard because the kid was studying a lot. A couple of years ago, I met him again, but he was no longer a child—he was already a movie producer with good vision in both eyes, sometimes dry, sometimes fatigued with some weak tendencies (which happens to anyone who uses their eyes too much), but with no absence of vision.

Your children are precious. More and more people want to learn from me how to work with them. The key is not to let other people trick you into giving up on your own children. First and foremost, don't listen to the optometrist who tells you that your child should adjust to eyeglasses. Glasses are like instruments: sometimes we have no choice but to wear them simply because education requires a lot of reading. But then, put them on and take them off as you study. That is true for adults as well as for children; it is especially critical for kids because those who keep wearing glasses will eventually have a great amount of nearsightedness. Therefore, the important thing is to use them as a tool, just like you use binoculars to see distance, or a telescope to look at stars, and not ever to use them as something that has to be a part of your face. This is extremely important. They are as addictive as drugs, as destructive as a bad habit, and a bad thing to do for your eyes. I would like to urge every parent and every responsible adult to have his or her child wear glasses only when the child gets tired of looking or doesn't see well. It is also relevant to find time to work with red-and-green glasses. Let the medical profession give up on your kids; you shouldn't.

I've been working with Lukas, who has an amblyopic eye (a lazy eye, 20/20 with one eye, 20/60 with the other) and does not use it. How very interested he was in that eye whenever he looked through the red-and-green glasses and saw pictures through the green lens. Then he stopped

being interested in seeing pictures and was only attracted to reading letters; then he was fascinated by art. It is essential to discover along with
your child—not just to tell him or her—what is interesting to the brain;
this will help to stimulate the weaker eye. You can't simply *do* an exercise
with a child, because a child develops the brain through curiosity. And one
of the most captivating things for both children and adults is that what
makes us curious at one moment in our life may not evoke our curiosity
at another time. For adults, what interests us presently might not interest
us in six months. For a child, what may have been interesting two days
ago may not be interesting now simply because of development. It is our
job to know what truly interests our children.

It's important to learn from your children what they want to see; you
cannot tell them what is going to interest them. I will never forget the
time my daughter went for a routine test and met an optometrist who
was not familiar to her. She was used to a very nice young man who,
in a very loving way, would measure her vision before her visit with
the ophthalmologist. At this point, however, there was a new optometrist: a woman who measured her vision, and my daughter immediately
saw worse. Consequently, the optometrist employed greater and greater
corrections, as they normally and very mistakenly do. Instead of my
daughter's vision being around 20/30 or 20/40, it became 20/100. When
I arrived at the hospital after that appointment and before the doctor's
appointment, I found my ex-wife very upset. I put my daughter on my
shoulders, gave her an eye patch to cover her left eye, and asked her to
look at the cars that were moving below the window of the seventh floor
at UCSF's hospital. It was a wonderful view, and she became extremely
interested in everything: the cars, the trees. Though I personally wasn't
interested in cars and trees, who am I to discourage someone, about to
be ten years old, who looked and looked and looked. I had to take a
break for a moment, and when I returned to the doctor's office, I discovered that her vision without glasses was 20/60—way better than the
20/100 with correction. And the doctor looked at her eyes and started
to joke with her, saying, "I see that you have boyfriends in your eyes."
And she yelled at him and said, "I have no boyfriends." He asked her
then, "What do you like to eat?" She said, "Pizza." He asked, "What do

you think about the pizza in the cafeteria here?" She said, "Pizza!" and she yelled at him like you would yell at a beloved uncle. He made a lot of money from her surgeries; she was an external patient. But the connection between them was very deep, and she was one of his most successful cases: a bright young kid whom he held in high regard while at the peak of his career. There was such a deep connection between them that when she was near him, she saw much better. The first time—three days before she turned ten—she saw 20/20 on the eye chart. His interest was piqued because I was there and I had put her on my shoulders. Her need to see better increased because she was there with a physician who wanted to see her at her best, who looked at it like an objective test he needed to pass; she cooperated because she wanted him to pass. Both of them had a unity and a union that neither was aware of. That's how you should feel as a parent: Encourage your child to see best just by being concerned.

I was able to stretch the interest in certain ways with my daughter for as long as three years, but no more than that. For ten years she wasn't interested in the waves near her home even when she was looking at them. She became interested in waves ten years later as she became a young woman. I had to find other ways to capture her interest, like putting her on my shoulders and taking her to the beach. Another way was going to a museum and getting her to close one eye while looking at different pictures.

The point is not only to evoke interest in your children, but also to be interested in the same things ourselves in order to best understand our children. And then, if there is an amblyopic eye, a strabismic (cross-sighted) eye, or a weak eye, to stimulate it. I was able to persuade my kids to be interested in clouds, rain, and signs, while they were blocking their strong eye with an obstructive lens and looking with their weak eye. I cannot tell everyone through this book what will interest their own children, which could be different things in different times. In Lukas's case, it was pictures at first, then letters, then art, and now we're waiting to see what's going to interest him next. The interest can also be the way in which we do things. For example, when I get my classes to sequentially put the small, medium, and large pieces of paper between their eyes and wave their hands to the side quickly, they are interested in it as a new exercise; however, their interest soon wanes. What then draws their attention is playing music and dancing and clapping hands with each other. As you can imagine, my classes become very dynamic. People stand up with a small piece of paper between their eyes and, looking at the paper, they clap each other's hands, seeing their hands and each other's hands in their periphery, which wakes up their periphery greatly. Next, they do the same with the medium piece of paper, then the large one, and then they repeat it with the medium and small pieces of paper. All of a sudden it seems that the small paper doesn't exist for them, because their periphery has become so wide, and when they remove the small paper, they don't understand how their field of vision has become so large. There is also a sense of more light in the room, even though there is not actually any additional light—it only seems that way because the retina receives so much more light in 90 percent of the people who have done this exercise. The Melissa Exercise can attract curiosity, and as I also mentioned, so can the Melissinia; the small piece of paper that you put on one eye is beneficial because the vision in that one eye expands.

Similar to children, adults also lose interest; however, children lose it first. As adults, it is our job not to fight with them, and not to demand from them, but to actually learn what gets them interested. I can vouch for my twenty-six-year-old son and twenty-three-year-old daughter, both of whom will take an interest in obstructing the strong eye (for my daughter, it is the left one; for my son, the right) and playing ball with each other for at least a short while. After five minutes, however, I'd better find something different because it will lose their interest, and I still want them to do the exercise. That's why we have invented so many exercises: to bring the curious mind into activity so that the eyes can function at their best, with the same principles we have brought to you through this book.

Sônia, who gave a wonderful acknowledgment and dedication to this book, is a relatively young practitioner of my work, as she's approaching her late forties. She was born and raised in Brazil and has been practicing for many years in a town called Rio Claro. In the past, when Brazil was still a Third World country, some generous donors from England had donated funds to build a special room specifically for Sônia's practice in Rio Claro. It's a dark room with many lights, swings, and computers. Sônia is well educated; she studied at four different universities and learned how to help the visually impaired use computers with both sound and large print. She also learned how to work with mentally challenged people and helped them reach the maximum of their capacity to function well in life. Sônia has also worked with deaf people. With her great work, people from all the region of São Paulo came to work with Sônia at the public clinic, to be helped by her to adjust to their disabilities and function well. But Sônia has never felt comfortable to simply help people adjust to being disabled; she always wants to find a way out of their limitations. This is probably because she had a very rough adolescence herself. She was sexually assaulted at gunpoint, but decided to help humanity, to help individuals move forward and be in a better place. This is a different attitude than many others who are assaulted. She became pregnant as a result of that assault and decided to keep the kid, which was a wonderful decision. That kid became a beautiful woman, a very good dentist, and a wonderful professional.

Sônia heard about my work as it became more known in Brazil and came to one of my big workshops. She approached an ophthalmologist who worked with her and had been sending people for her to train to function with their disabilities and to reach their potential. She asked him to come with her to the workshop, but he said that I must be a charlatan. He wasn't the first or the last to say that, but I hadn't heard that for a long time. I heard it in my adolescence and lately I've heard it only once, during a talk show in Berkeley, California. Sônia brought the ophthalmologist to my workshop, and he was so impressed that at the end of the workshop, he bought all of my literature. She then decided to attend training in my work, and eventually became a trainer. While the apprenticeship program or intern program takes 500 hours, she studied for 1,500 hours. Everything that Sônia does, she does in a deep way. And so you can assume that any time that she meets a person in need, she has a great desire to help. Which is what happened to Maria.

Maria came crying to the public clinic that Sônia was running. It was the same clinic that started with donations from England and became one of the most famous public clinics in South America, thanks to Sônia.

Maria was sent by an ophthalmologist because her four-month-old infant was born without an iris, which was a disaster. The iris does many things for the eye: it expands the diameter of the pupil and shrinks it; it expands for night vision and shrinks for day vision. Also, the pupils, to a great extent, affect your sense of well-being just as the autonomic nervous system that puts you on alert or puts you in a place of relaxation is affected by pupillary diameter. And the pupils, to a great extent, determine how much light will get into your retina. It affects your nervous system. The ophthalmologist said to the mother, "This baby is not going to see. She's going to be blind." So when Maria came to Sônia she said, "My baby is going to be blind for life." Sônia looked at the baby. She understood the feeling of the ophthalmologist, but she experimented for herself, as she always does. She is an explorer. She shined light in the infant's eye and she saw that the infant was responding. She looked at the mom with a great sense of concern and said, "Can you imagine the possibility that your baby will not be blind?" The mother was startled. "Of course not. The ophthalmologist said she'll be blind."

Sônia knew that at that age, a mother and a daughter are one unit; nothing truly separates them, and their skin is nothing but a connective tissue between them. Sônia felt a great affinity with the mother and connected to her situation. Her eyes were asking the mother to look at a different possibility and a different reality, and their connection was heart to heart. She then asked, "Would you imagine the possibility that your baby can see?" The mother said, "Maybe. Maybe she won't be blind after all." And then Sônia taught her sunning and how to palm her daughter, as well as massaging, light therapy, blinking light in the dark, and all the therapies that she learned from me. Only she did them better. The mother came back again and again, and after four months, a full, normal iris was formed. The ophthalmologist said, "I don't understand this." And Sônia showed it to me with great relief and with tears. I looked into Sônia's soul and I told myself this is how the world should be.

Chapter 8

The Blind Spots
of Conventional Wisdom

The Hidden Danger of Sunglasses

It has become common for people in our culture to immediately put on sunglasses as soon as they step out of the house on a sunny day. People see the sun as some sort of enemy that is about to cause harm to their eyes. Doctors warn us of the dangers of sun exposure, and there certainly are reasons to take the proper precautions to protect our bodies from too much exposure to ultraviolet light. Our eyes, however, are made to function at their highest and best when they are exposed to a full range of light and darkness.

It's important to be in touch with our bodies on a cellular level. You can't normally see your cells unless you have microscopic pictures taken of them and are able to look at the pictures. We tend to ignore our body and our body parts. But it is very important to have a very thorough feel for our own body.

Enjoy the sun and also the dark of night. Hardly ever wear sunglasses because they weaken the pupils. Enjoy the sun throughout the day, and don't use a flashlight when you take a walk at night. Enjoy the expansion of the pupils at night. Make your eyes more vital and more alive. Give your eyes a sense of love so that, in many ways, you love your life and you love the universe. Allow your eyes to develop good fixation, which is the ability to allow the proper amount of light to enter the pupils in order to see better in whatever situation you are in. When your pupils become firmer and not sluggish, you can then have a better fixation, and allow the exact amount of light you need for your sight to improve.

In the daytime, you will end up seeing details in much greater clarity. This will take the load and distress away from other parts of the visual system, like the retina and the lens. At nighttime, your pupils will be wide enough to see all that is around you in the dark. Your whole system will become stronger as a result of your pupils being able to absorb more light.

Ignoring your eyes, not giving them enough darkness or enough light, weakens the system through the years. Renewing our strength by reducing the amount of time we wear sunglasses, and reducing the amount of time we spend indoors, can make a huge difference. Be wary of the sun scare.

Many people do not realize that we have pigments in our eyes that darken the light. It's called the melanin pigment, which is in the choroid area, the area that nourishes the retina. One of the ten layers of the retina is melanin, so the retina itself has a whole layer of pigment that darkens the light. Therefore, you have "sunglasses" inside the retina itself. When you wear sunglasses, it reduces the usefulness of the melanin layer, and the body will produce less melanin. It also darkens the light as it arrives at the retina, so you do not use your own pigments to darken the light. Consequently, your pigments migrate to the back of the retina, less of it is produced for the retina and for the skin, and they are not as effective as they could have been otherwise.

Believe it or not, sunglasses hurt your retina just as much as crutches can hurt one's legs. If your legs were weak and you were quick in using a cane or crutches or braces to walk with, you may never give up your crutches. But if you worked very hard on strengthening your legs, there is a possibility you would regain their full use. In some cases there isn't such a possibility, and that's when crutches or braces are very useful. If there were such a possibility, and you could strengthen your legs, you wouldn't use crutches as a method of healing, since it's best to work on the body's independence.

The same is true for sunglasses. The more you use sunglasses, the weaker your pupils become. You also are weakening your defense mechanism that has existed in your retina and in your ancestors' retinas for millions of years. What's more, when you wear sunglasses, you produce less melanin, which then affects your skin as well as your eyes. I have heard of research showing how a couple of villages of Australian Aborigines were informed by the medical profession that they must wear sunglasses, and it was the first time in their history they got sunburned as a consequence. The reason is when you do not produce enough melanin, it's a systemic issue. We need to produce enough melanin to protect ourselves from the sun, to darken the light. It's like the paper that a photographer uses to decrease light intensity in the photography shop. The same thing happens with melanin. It darkens the light, and therefore the light can concentrate better in the retina. Wearing sunglasses does the work of our own pigments, and so we produce less of them. But that production affects your skin and also affects your mood, because without good light, it's hard for almost any human to be in a good mood.

I live in a city that many people like to leave occasionally because of the fog. There are people who live in Seattle, where there's a lot of rain, and others in Scandinavia, many of whom are very depressed because they don't have enough light. We need the light to be much less depressed because it actually induces chemical activity, like release of serotonin. The light combines with hemoglobin and creates an amazing buildup—which some people are saying is similar to photosynthesis—that releases serotonin, and the serotonin leads to optimism. There is no medication—including Prozac or any other antidepressant—that can make you as optimistic as sunlight, if you absorb it properly.

If you practice sunning for at least twenty minutes a day, you will find that your eyes adjust much better to the sun. The sun, throughout the years, will become very comfortable for you. You will also find that darkness is easier for you to handle. The dark will not appear to be as dark, as your pupils grow wider and your retinal cells get more sensitive. Best of all, you will enjoy widely opening your eyes in both the strongest and the weakest light. You will also be happier because the combination of the sun's rays and the hemoglobin in the blood releases many hormones and neurotransmitters, like serotonin, that lead to a sense of joy. You will probably also have an easier time releasing melatonin at night without taking any vitamins or drugs, simply because of your good sun exposure. The joy of this will lead to many other good things in your life.

If your eyes are sun-sensitive and do not widen enough in the dark, the other mechanisms, even if they're healthy, may not function to the best of their potential. Most of what the visual system does is absorbing light and processing it. Therefore, it's important that that process be easy and relaxing for the body.

Dangers of Corrective Lenses

There are three essential dangers from utilizing corrective lenses. If you wear glasses, you tend not to use as much of your external muscles because you depend on a focal point. They also cause us not to pay attention to the periphery, because we normally look within their frame. For this reason, you weaken the eyes through the years, which is very bad for your total mechanism.

If you wear contact lenses, your body wants to reject them at first because they are foreign objects. This means you must weaken the immune system in your eyes in order to accept the contacts. This weakens the entire eye over time. Also, the contacts prevent enough oxygen from coming to the eyes, because the contact lenses block it. Even the permeable contact lenses are not permeable enough for oxygen, and they are hard to clean.

And whether you wear glasses or contacts, the biggest danger is simply the sense of dependency you create. The more you wear them, the more you need them. You never give your eyes the chance to work out and to regain their sense of strength and natural ability.

At the age of forty-five, seven out of eight people wear corrective lenses. I don't think we were ever born to have all this correction. The reason that we have all this correction is that we are creatures of imitation. There are many millions of brain cells that only work to imitate each other. Monkeys imitate each other, and humans imitate other humans. By practicing vision improvement and being adamant about it, you will be able to affect your vision and the world for the better. This book will change the world completely because many boundaries will break in what we believe our real capacity is. Just imagine how many diseases will be prevented as a result of people working on their eyes.

Now you know how to measure your own vision. You have an eye chart on the wall. Let's assume that you read the fourth line with great ease, and then you read the fifth, sixth, and seventh with more difficulty. By the eighth, you can't read anymore. If this is true, you're standing exactly in the right place. It could be three, five, ten, or twenty feet.

Now also determine five or six different objects in your environment that you like to look at. These objects could be flowers from three yards away, or a fence from a yard or two. Changeable items like the clouds in the sky cannot measure your improvement, but steady objects, with steady light at the same time of day, can.

When you reduce your prescription and first see with a weaker prescription, just be aware of the fact that you will not see as well initially. Normally, within three weeks you will improve. Keep the glasses in your pocket all the time, but try to see well without them as long as it feels effortless. Don't squint or strain. Just look softly through the fog or fuzziness you have, and work on your mind to reduce your frustration.

The most important thing to remember is that how we train ourselves to look is more important, for the time being, than what we see. With time, what we see will be more important. You're returning to the process of looking. When you were an infant, you didn't see things well and you didn't care, because you didn't know that things could be seen any better than how you saw them. As you looked at details, from one to the other, your vision got better. Your macula, the *fovea centralis* inside it, and even the foveola, which is a smaller spot within the fovea that sees details, started to act well because your mind was interested in what you were looking at. As a result, the brain-and-eye connection became stronger. Slowly, as you started to crawl and walk, the brain developed, and the eyes became stronger, seeing better and better. Normally, childhood vision is so much better than adult vision. Many people measure childhood vision as 20/15, which is better than 20/20. We want to return to that phase. We want to look with great curiosity at all the details the world gives us. Some are nice and some are ugly, but we always want to look.

One woman who had started to lose her vision stated in one of my classes, "I stopped having any interest in looking at things because, in my opinion, the city I live in is ugly." I could understand why she stopped looking at details, but the more we look consciously at details, the better we see them. There are many people who live in beautiful cities like San Francisco and still do not look at details. Remember: all details, whether beautiful or not, can be interesting. Remember that when you were an infant, all details were interesting to you.

Looking through your fog could be interesting as well. For example, you can look at the different details in flowers from a distance where you can see the flowers relatively well; then look away, either at a fence, a bush, the sky, or buildings that are farther away, but you still see some details in them. Close your eyes and visualize the contrast between details at a far distance. You can visualize the leaf of a bush and the sky, the fence and the earth, or whatever has different contrasts. Then look at the objects again, and return to the flowers. Many people see the flowers better.

Straining your eyes to look far makes you see worse; looking far without strain, with the help of your imagination, and with the help of seeing more and more details, allows you to see better from nearby. Nearsighted people need to work on slowly making the point of focus farther away. This means a nearsighted person who sees really well from eight inches should hope that, after beginning this practice, he or she will see really well from ten, then twelve inches. It is the ability to see farther and farther at a distance, even if it is from a relatively close range, that is going to heal your myopia.

So, the number one thing to remember is, when you put your glasses in your pocket, don't worry about identifying people's faces. Announce to all your friends, relatives, and family that, right now, you have decided to spend the next four to six months using your glasses as little as possible in order to improve your vision problems. The main thing is to make sure that when you look at the world, you look at the world from the eyes with which you were born. Make sure that you blink. Adjust to the world as it is. Enjoy it.

Keep in mind that, if your tendency is to wear glasses, you can improve your vision enough that glasses won't be necessary. In fact, you may end up seeing better without them than you had originally been seeing with them. If you have recovered from a major eye surgery with rehabilitation, instead of just seeing the top of the chart with your glasses, you may see the bottom of the chart with your glasses. If you cannot recover your vision, you may learn how to use the little vision that you have to function as fully as you can with your eyes and body. There is a possibility for rehabilitation in every situation, and we need to believe in our eyes to create such a revolution. This revolution will come from the simple truth that we have inner powers and that this book has helped you to reach them. With diligence, faith, love, and work, we will be able to change ourselves and all who are around us, until this world is a better place.

As I have pointed out, the medical establishment has few answers for most of our common eye disorders. Even so, it is important to ask: if reliable and safe treatments *did* exist, who would pay for them?

It is my opinion that the time has come for all of us to ask what the real cost of vision problems is, not just in terms of money, but also in terms of productivity, quality of life, and morale. When someone loses their eyesight, their entire life is affected, along with the lives of everyone they know. It isn't just their problem, it is society's problem. The reality of it is that by neglecting each other, we neglect ourselves—and, in the end, we all pay dearly.

I hope we all realize that the expense for vision care is exponential and continues to grow; it is very hard to meet it with the money we currently have, and it will cost even more in the future. While we try to cover costs with local, state, and federal budgets, the study of extensive ophthalmology—with all the specialized equipment it involves—is more costly than any level of government can handle. To concentrate on any one particular area in this field involves that much more time and money.

Sadly, there is no help coming from the medical profession to reinforce strength in the eyes. We need to find natural ways to strengthen the eyes so we can see better, and depend less on ophthalmology so that it will be less costly to the community. Most people harbor the false belief that their eyes cannot get better. Therefore, we need to start with new seeds of hope until more people in the world are willing to work on their eyes. In fact, we need a silent but continuous revolution. This goes beyond countries or flags. To believe in ourselves and in our eyes is to open a window to the heart. With continuous work on the eyes, we can make a huge difference in our self-image and in resolving many other problems, personal or impersonal, national or international.

Positive reinforcement comes with positive results. Think about it: we relinquished our power to acute care, which is a false promise for the health of our eyes; when you do so for one problem, the next one often appears rather quickly. The truth is that if we ourselves took good care of our eyes, the few times that we needed acute care would work just fine and we would also rehabilitate more quickly.

Because physicians think that nothing can be fixed in the eye except by the mechanical acute care of which they're capable, they are not researching the vital forces of the eyes; however, we have several vital forces. We have the macula that, when linked properly with the brain through our shifting exercises, will start to be more active while keeping its vigilance, vitality, and strength. We have our minds that, through imagery and memory, can reinforce much better vision. We have our lenses that, when we balance their use, become much more flexible. We have our pupils that, if they contract much in the daylight and expand much at nighttime, become stronger. We can also have good circulation with which we can improve our eyes, refresh them, and prevent most vision-related problems from happening with age.

The truth of the matter is that it's very important to create great internal changes. Sometimes this requires that you change or widen your whole being. You can acquire new skills that you didn't have before, ones that are exciting and useful to you. These may be skills of any kind. There are more than 87,000 professions on earth. In the near future, there could be over 100,000 professions. Even if you don't change your profession, you could learn new ways of operating and functioning. If you change your profession, do it with grace and ease. Another important thing is that many people are already at the end of their careers. They have accomplished their goals at work by the age of forty-five or fifty. It is wonderful to see so many of these people, who are in their forties, fifties, and sixties, returning to schools all over the world to acquire new knowledge and skills.

It is important on an emotional level that you have something to look forward to in life, that you feel your life is meaningful, and that every moment of your life is creative. This emotional advancement is the background of healing. It's hard to heal if you resent your own life. It is easier to heal if you feel that you have something to look forward to. In this way you can help others and yourself at the same time. It motivates you to invest in the time it takes to improve your vision. It gives you the vigilance to maintain your improvement as time goes on. It gives you the impetus to feel well enough within yourself to change for the better.

Your happiness is precious. It comes with self-acceptance, and there is no better time than in your forties, fifties, and sixties to work on self-acceptance. When we have self-acceptance, we place less importance on adding extra weight or on the wrinkles that come with age. This is a time when we like all we've done, all we are currently doing, and all we will be doing. Believe me, our beauty will reflect itself. A straight face with no wrinkles does not match a wrinkled face with great happiness. A thin and fit Hollywood body is not nearly as attractive as an energetic body, even if it appears to be imperfect. At this particular time in life, working on a sense of inner happiness and working on a particular part of our body are parallel goals. Working on our flexibility and devoting ourselves to expanding our thoughts are comparable to each other. Slowly but surely, your vision will get better and better. If you keep shifting and looking at details, you will maintain the vigilance of thought and the emotional openness required. This kind of maturity is our next step in life.

So, what we need is to inform ourselves, to work with ourselves, to convince others, to suggest support groups, and to suggest change in the world, bringing it to the consciousness of everyone we meet. Explain to them that it's time for us to be aware of our powers. Who knows—maybe as a result of what you do, new research will spring up in your home town and it will make this a much better world than the one we currently live in. Because, unlike what most people believe, our world is not as developed as it could be. Our eyes, so precious to us, could see so much better along with those of every human being on earth. I'm the one to tell you that. I could be blind right now, but I can read this book. And why? Simply because I worked on myself.

This is why it is more important than ever to spread the word that it is possible for us to take care of our own vision. It can be done in such a way that we never develop devastating eye problems in the first place, thus never having to rely on the inadequate and antiquated approaches of our governments or of the corporate medical establishment.

The way to solve the crisis of low- or no-budget vision care is to heal our eyes ourselves. Learn the basic exercises in *Vision for Life*. Become aware of the erosive habits you may be developing from staring at a computer screen all day and a television screen all night. Learn to blink. Learn to breathe correctly. Learn to relax. Learn to give massages so you and your loved ones can help each other maintain good blood flow along with a relaxed, confident, and radiant state of being.

This is the path to a sustainable future for our eyes. This is my vision for life.

Index

Acknowledgments

I began this book by speaking into a cassette recorder, and what I said was transcribed word for word onto paper. To translate from the spoken word into written material is not easy, and, in fact, my dictation was not something easily conveyed in words, something pictorial and easily described; it was more like lyrical prose, and needed a lot of work in order to become a comprehensive tool for the reader. Yet, when I considered all the wonderful people my method had enabled me to help and the exciting new discoveries they had experienced, and when I thought about the hope I wanted to give to billions of people in the world along with my own patients, with the help of many, I began the real work of putting a book together. Therefore, I thank Phillip Barcio for helping to compile the materials and making my ideas more comprehensible. Next, I would very much like to thank my friend Richard Mandrachio, whose talents as an editor helped enormously in presenting the book in a straightforward manner that all readers can understand and practice with. I also wish to give many thanks to photographer Richard Miller, who himself benefited tremendously from this work; he improved his vision in spite of a birth defect and a condition that caused major loss of his optic nerve. He regained much of his vision and, through black and white pictures, was able to bring to life many of the exercises that will help you, the reader. The person to whom I extend heartfelt gratitude more than anyone else is my good friend Jan Albin, who worked tirelessly for countless hours on all the forms the manuscript has taken. Jan offered an incredible amount of aid in editing this book and was instrumental in getting it published. I would further like to thank the staff at the School for Self-Healing for their assistance in the writing process and their contributions, both large and small, that helped bring this book to publication. Finally, my sincere thanks go to the editors and good people at North Atlantic Books who accepted my manuscript for publication.

About the Author

Born blind, **MEIR SCHNEIDER** taught himself to see and over forty years has developed a pioneering program of healing and recovery for the sighted and the blind. Despite many obstacles he has pushed his work worldwide and is now acknowledged and recognized by most natural vision improvement practitioners in the world. Named one of the ten most inspirational people of Israel by a top national Israeli news program, Schneider is the founder and head teacher of the School for Self-Healing in San Francisco, which offers programs that satisfy the continuing education requirements of the American Massage Therapy Association (AMTA), the California Board of Registered Nursing, and the National Certification Board for Therapeutic Massage and Bodywork (NCBTMB). The School for Self-Healing has helped hundreds of thousands of people seeking solutions to chronic health conditions, including many people with vision problems. Schneider shares his remarkable results not only at the School for Self-Healing and at programs worldwide, but also in popular books, CDs, and DVDs.

About North Atlantic Books

North Atlantic Books (NAB) is a 501(c)(3) nonprofit publisher committed to a bold exploration of the relationships between mind, body, spirit, culture, and nature. Founded in 1974, NAB aims to nurture a holistic view of the arts, sciences, humanities, and healing. To make a donation or to learn more about our books, authors, events, and newsletter, please visit www.northatlanticbooks.com.